Health Care Chaplaincy in Oncology

Health Care Chaplaincy in Oncology

Laurel Arthur Burton, ThD
George Handzo, MDiv
Editors

The Haworth Pastoral Press
An Imprint of The Haworth Press, Inc.
New York • London • Norwood (Australia)

Published by

The Haworth Pastoral Press, 10 Alice Street, Binghamton, NY 13904-1580 USA

The Haworth Pastoral Press is an Imprint of The Haworth Press, Inc., 10 Alice Street, Binghamton, NY 13904-1580 USA.

Health Care Chaplaincy in Oncology has also been published as *Journal of Health Care Chaplaincy*, Volume 4, Numbers 1/2 1992.

Library of Congress Cataloging-in-Publication Data

Health care chaplaincy in oncology / Laurel Arthur Burton, George Handzo, editors.
     p. cm.
     "Also . . . published as Journal of health care chaplaincy, volume 4, numbers 1/2, 1992."
     Includes bibliographical references and index.
     ISBN 1-56024-200-0 (alk. paper)
     1. Pastoral medicine. 2. Chaplains, Hospital. 3. Cancer–Patients–Pastoral counseling of. 4. Church work with the sick. I. Burton, Laurel Arthur. II. Handzo, George.
BV4335.H33   1992
259'.4–dc20
                                                                          92-25898
                                                                             CIP

ABOUT THE EDITORS

Laurel Arthur Burton, ThD, FCOC, is Bishop Anderson Professor of Religion and Medicine at Rush University, Rush-Presbyterian-St. Luke's Medical Center in Chicago, Illinois, where he serves as Chairman of the Department of Religion, Health, and Human Values. Dr. Burton also directs and teaches in the university's humanities program as well as teaching and supervising marriage and family therapy in the Department of Psychiatry. He is also a member of the Ethics Consultation Service. He is currently Senior Editor of *The CareGiver Journal* for the College of Chaplains, and has authored or edited seven books and over thirty articles. Twice a graduate of Boston University, Dr. Burton was an administrator and teacher at the B.U. Medical Center, then at Harvard Divinity School prior to moving to Rush-Presbyterian-St. Luke's Medical Center. He is married and lives in Chicago with his wife and two almost grown children.

George Handzo, MDiv, FCOC, came to Memorial Sloan-Kettering in 1978 as Pediatric Chaplain and is now also Director of the Chaplaincy Service. He is on the staff of The Hospital Chaplaincy, Inc., of New York City. Rev. Handzo was educated at Princeton University and Yale University Divinity School and also holds a second masters degree in Educational Psychology. Rev. Handzo is a member of the National Clergy Task Force of the American Cancer Society, and has lectured widely and written on issues such as talking with children about death and loss and chaplaincy with oncology patients. He also serves on the National Education Committee of the College of Chaplains, Inc. Rev. Handzo is married and the father of two young children. One of his most remarkable accomplishments is that he is a Licensed Soccer Coach.

ABOUT THE CONTRIBUTORS

Gordon P. Beam was ordained in the Free Gospel Church almost 35 years ago. He has taught, served parishes, and is a volunteer chaplain at Dover General Hospital in Dover, NJ.

Laurel Arthur Burton is Bishop Anderson Professor of Religion and Medicine and Chairman of the Department of Religion, Health, and Human Values at Rush-Presbyterian-St. Luke's Medical Center in Chicago, IL. He is a Fellow in the College of Chaplains and a Clinical Member of the American Association for Marriage and Family Therapy. He also holds the designation of Approved Supervisor from the AAMFT.

David F. Cella is Director of the Division of Psychosocial Oncology, and an Associate Professor at Rush-Presbyterian-St. Luke's Medical Center.

Elaine Goodell is a Certified Chaplain and Fellow of the College of Chaplains. She is on the staff of The Hospital Chaplaincy, Inc. of New York City and the Chaplaincy Service at Memorial Sloan-Kettering Cancer Center.

George Handzo is a Certified Chaplain and Fellow in the College of Chaplains. He is on the staff of The Hospital Chaplaincy, Inc. of New York City and Director of the Chaplaincy Service at Memorial Sloan-Kettering Cancer Center.

Jimmie C. Holland is Chief of the Psychiatry Service at Memorial Sloan-Kettering Cancer Center in New York City.

Daniel G. O'Hare is Fellow-in-Ethics in the Psychiatry Service at Memorial Sloan-Kettering Cancer Center in New York City.

Mary T. O'Neill is an ACPE and NACC Supervisor and Director of Pastoral Services at Calvary Hospital in the Bronx, NY.

Mark Peterson is the Director of Pastoral Care at Bayfront Medical Center in St. Petersburg, FL.

Jeffery Silberman is a Rabbi and CPE Supervisor. He is on the staff of The Hospital Chaplaincy, Inc. of New York City and Co-Director of the Department of Pastoral Care at Lenox Hill Hospital.

Avery D. Weisman is Senior Psychiatrist at Massachusetts General Hospital in Boston, MA.

The Editors also wish to acknowledge the tireless, volunteer services of Elaine Ingstrom who typed the entire manuscript.

Health Care Chaplaincy in Oncology

CONTENTS

∞   ALL THE HAWORTH PASTORAL PRESS
BOOKS AND JOURNALS ARE PRINTED
ON CERTIFIED ACID-FREE PAPER

Introduction

"If it hadn't been for you, we never would have survived all this," said the man. He could have been talking to a doctor or a nurse or any one of several healthcare professionals. In fact, he was talking to the chaplain who had been a faithful companion through his wife's multiple hospitalizations. She had been diagnosed with breast cancer and treated aggressively. Later a bone marrow transplant had been a seemingly last ditch, experimental effort. At the time of her discharge, the patient was doing well and her husband was grateful. "Everyone was great, but having your support, your quiet presence and prayers, was really important. Thanks."

From the earliest days of religious communities, religious and spiritual advisors have been important in the companioning of people in the midst of trouble. They have been *keystones of care*. Jews were admonished not to live far from a physician and observed the mitzva to visit the sick. Christians established centers of hospitality to care for the sick and the poor. In traditional culture caring and healing were (and are) linked with religious and spiritual practice.

Cancer is one of the most dread diagnoses in the medical arena. "Will you pray for my sister? She's just gotten a diagnosis of cancer and you know what that means." In fact, we never know exactly what that means. A diagnosis of cancer does *not* mean just one thing. Some cancers are marvelously treatable, while others, inexplicably, are less so. Still, the fears of patients, families and friends alike are profoundly real.

"Pray for a miracle, will you chaplain?" Most of us in pastoral care do believe in miracles of one sort or another. They don't have to be spectacular, spontaneous healings. Often, miracles are experienced in terms of healing of the spirit, amazing demonstrations of courage, abiding expressions of love. Some of us wonder, still, what can and should we pray for? What *is* possible? What can we do? How do we balance active interventions with faithful presence?

More than that, what does it mean to be a person of faith in the midst of ministry to people with cancer?

This book began with a conference at Memorial Sloan-Kettering Cancer Center. Most of the people who attended were members of the clergy or religious orders who regularly work with oncology patients. Many expressed a clear need for more written resources. As we began to work on the manuscript, however, we found places where we wanted more. Occasional chapters were added to fill-out the original picture. We've divided this volume into several sections.

We begin with *What Pastoral Care Providers Should Know About Cancer.* Here Gordon Beam, a member of the College of Chaplains who has experienced cancer first hand, reminds us of the fears that accompany the diagnosis. His testimony to the power and importance of human support and prayer ground pastoral care in the reality of spiritual experience. Next, Jimmie Holland, Chief of Psychiatry at Memorial Sloan-Kettering in New York City, provides a clear and concise introduction to the topic of cancer risk and survival. Since there is evidence that religious people often seek the advice of trusted spiritual advisors, pastoral care professionals may be in a position to encourage healthy lifestyles, early detection, and improved quality of life during treatment.

The next three chapters, under the general heading of *Providers of Care* include reflections on the role of spiritual counselors by psychiatrist Avery Weisman, and chaplains George Handzo and Jeffery Silberman. Their insights shed light on the special identity and calling of pastoral care providers (and their relationship to and with God) in the midst of work with oncology patients.

The following two chapters deal with *Pastoral Care of Families with Cancer.* Larry Burton, a chaplain and family therapist, takes a systems approach and claims that the patient is the whole family, not just the one with the physician diagnosis. He surveys family therapy theories and suggests some useful tools for chaplains. Elaine Goodell writes of her experience with a particular family and through her narrative evokes the power of the particular relationship of chaplain and patient/family.

The final section is devoted to *Special Concerns.* First, psychologist David Cella outlines specific techniques chaplains and other clinicians may use in promoting "wellness" among cancer patients. Then, Mary T. O'Neill focuses on the special characteristics of caring when the patient is at the end of his/her length of days. Daniel O'Hare provides an insightful and care-full discussion of the care provider's moral voice in the cancer process, and Mark Peterson describes a practical model for training local clergy to minister more effectively with people who have cancer.

Futurists John Naisbitt and Patricia Aburdene claim that "Science and technology do not tell us what life means. We learn that through literature, the arts, and spirituality."[1] When people are faced with the prospect of cancer, it is no surprise that they turn to both medicine and spirituality. Medicine offers hope for troubled bodies while spirituality offers hope for anxious selves. The role of pastoral care providers in the midst of a diagnosis of cancer is perhaps, now more than ever, a *keystone of care.*

Laurel Arthur Burton, ThD
Chicago, IL

George Handzo, MDiv
New York, NY

NOTE

1. Naisbitt, J. and Aburdene, P. (1990) *Megatrends 2000.* New York: Avon Books. p. 293.

WHAT PASTORAL CARE PROVIDERS SHOULD KNOW ABOUT CANCER

A First-Hand Encounter with Cancer

Gordon P. Beam, BTh

"God knows the way that I take . . ." (Job 23:10) I have always found these words helpful; so have many of the patients at the hospital where I serve as a volunteer chaplain. However these words became an unbelievable source of strength to *me* as I faced cancer in my own life.

For several months I had noticed, but ignored, the warning signs: weight loss, exhaustion after brief sessions of work, small, hard tumors surfacing in different parts of my body. Finally my wife and daughter prevailed upon me to see a doctor. At first he didn't seem to be very concerned, but after ordering blood work found that my electrolytes were grossly out of range and that I had a highly elevated CPK. This doctor referred me to a rheumatologist. After many more tests including chest x-rays, EMG, barium swallow x-rays, more blood work, the rheumatologist couldn't make a diagnosis either. He decided I must have a muscular disease and wanted to have a portion of muscle removed from my upper leg. He seemed to ignore the tumors, especially those on the underside of my arm between the armpit and the elbow. My wife was not as confident as the doctor and urged him to remove the tumor from my arm for analysis. "Just to reassure me," she said. Reluctantly the doctor consented and the tumors were removed. Two weeks later the surgeon called to advise me that it was impossible to make a firm conclusion, but that "It is 95% sure that this is a lymphoma."

Contact was made with a major, urban cancer institute. The physician there examined me, re-examined the cold tumor tissue, and did more blood work. That blood work revealed a high titre for Epstein Barr Virus (EBV), the virus that causes mononucleosis among other things. This revealed that I am one of those less fortunate individuals with Chronic Epstein Barr Virus, and apparently this had been a problem since childhood. At least we were relieved that the "Big C" wasn't my problem. The doctor sent me on my way to eat well and get plenty of rest. "You should be fine," he said.

A year passed. My status changed only slightly. Now there were two more hard tumors on my upper arm. Again my wife was concerned and insisted that they be removed and analyzed. The doctor was reluctant since he was sure it wasn't cancer. We persisted and the tumors were removed. This time the lab results indicated Lymphoma (non-Hodgkins) in the advanced stage (Stage IV). Such news, delivered over the phone, left me devastated. As a chaplain I had dealt with patients receiving this kind of news, but now it was me.

I went to my first visit with the oncologist feeling numb. As I sat waiting my turn I observed others also waiting. One had no hair. Would this be me in a few weeks, I wondered? Others were experiencing severe nausea. Would I have to deal with this? One looked hopeless. Since my cancer was already in Stage IV I wondered if the doctor could help me? Would I die?

The doctor's words were reassuring. Lymph cancer, especially my type, was usually curable. The chemotherapy would be very strong, however. After my first treatment I felt some of the side effects almost immediately. I didn't know if I could get through all that I knew the coming months would hold. A nurse friend met my wife and I at the doctor's office. She brought encouragement and some homemade soup. At home, a friend called to tell me she was praying for my recovery. As the days passed, get well cards flooded in, along with notes and phone calls. Each assured me of prayerful support.

I remained strong and continued to work during the first two weeks of treatment. Then came the two weeks without treatments and I felt great. OK, I thought. I *can* do it. However, at the return to chemotherapy I began a swift down-hill slide and ended up in the hospital on Mother's Day. I had a violent headache and had spiked a temperature. I spent seven days there, undergoing multiple tests including a spinal tap to rule out viral meningitis. I was getting IV antibiotics, too, but I only got worse. Finally I was discharged from the hospital simply because I was so compromised from the treatment and illness that I was too apt to pick-up another infection.

It was obvious now that I would not be able to return to work, at least not for the duration of the chemotherapy. I hit bottom. My liver went into complete failure and I was jaundiced with terrible itching all over my body, no saliva, no fluid in my eyes. It was awful. Yet, somehow, I began to notice that I was acquiring a new attitude. Even though I wanted to be well and working, I was at peace. Somehow I felt lifted up by the prayer support of my friends from all over the world. I still asked "Why me," but now I heard an inner voice responding "Trust me." I did just that. I learned to lean on God.

Treatments stopped and I waited for three months for my liver to begin functioning again. When it did the chemotherapy began again. This time it was less aggressive, but still effective. Eight months passed. The only adverse reaction I had this time was a severe case of shingles down the left side of my neck, over my shoulder and onto my chest. During all this time I continued to receive cards, calls, and messages of encouragement. It meant so much. I was reminded of my CPE supervisor urging us to take note of the patient's surroundings when entering a room. He would ask, "Are there cards, flowers, plants, etc., that suggest a support system?" Now I knew why that was so important. Knowing that people really cared and prayed, and that I felt their prayers, held me strong during those months of recovery.

When I felt well enough I visited other sick people, even those with cancer. One of my first experiences was a man critically ill and facing chemotherapy. I found myself reliving it all, even to feeling the waves of nausea, as he described his treatments. His wife often introduced me to family and friends as "the chaplain who has cancer, too." She seemed to be observing both my wife and I to see how we were dealing with my illness. I wondered if we were unknowing models for her. Even our daughter, a nurse, experienced first hand the difference of dealing with cancer in one's own family instead of just with patients.

One day, as I entered the Chaplain's Office at the hospital where I volunteer, the secretary seemed to be holding back tears. When I asked about her, she quickly shared her news. That very morning she learned that her 22 year-old son had lymphoma. "Will he die?" she asked. I couldn't answer that question, of course, but I was able to share my personal experience with her, and assure her of my prayers and presence. She still had tears in her eyes when she said, "God sent you here today, just when I needed you."

The time arrived for another unpleasant bone marrow test to determine whether or not I was in remission. When the doctor called to say "It's good, you're in remission," you can imagine my joy. I was ecstatic! And I was grateful to God who had brought me through this difficult battle.

From time to time I had difficulty, like Job, finding God in my suffering. I knew what Job meant when he said, "I go forward, but God is not there; and backward, but I cannot perceive God: On the left hand where God works, but I cannot behold God. God hides on the right hand that I cannot see God" (Job 23:8-9). Because of the support of friends, colleagues, and family, through it all, when I didn't know how to find God, I was still able to be sure that God was there and that "God knows the way that I take . . ." Job 23:10

Can I Help Myself?
What Are the Psychological
and Social Factors
in Cancer Risk and Survival?

Jimmie C. Holland, MD

INTRODUCTION

The role of behavioral and psychosocial factors in cancer cause and survival has become an area of research since the 1950's. However, folk medicine beliefs have existed for a far longer period as a reaction to the intense fears of cancer, its stigma and the need to attribute cause to a frightening, incurable disease. In fact, the American Cancer Society was formed in 1913 to provide education about cancer to change the fatalistic attitudes and reverse the primary behavior which altered outcome: delay of individuals with suspicious symptoms in seeking medical consultation, which in turn resulted in less detection of early curable disease.[14] Many early studies of psychosocial variables explored the psychological issues and attitudes which contributed to delay.[15] The recognition of the line between lung cancer and cigarette smoking started a major effort in prevention and cancer control research which has expanded over the past decade into community education demonstration studies. Education to reduce cancer risk from exposures and life style has been impressive, as evidenced by the present concern about diet

Adapted with permission of the author from Psychosocial variables: Are they factors in cancer risk and survival? In Current Concepts in Psycho-Oncology IV, Syllabus, (1991) Eds. MJ Massie and L. Lesko, Memorial Sloan-Kettering Cancer Center, New York, NY.

and sun exposure. These efforts have largely been carried out by investigators in cancer prevention, cancer control and epidemiology.

A parallel research effort has developed since the fifties which has explored the psychological, social and behavioral factors in cancer morbidity and mortality. The early studies suffered from methodological weaknesses and unavailability of valid tools. Today, however, the use of more carefully designed studies and reliable assessment instruments have resulted in explosion of well conducted studies assessing the psychosocial variables. More recent studies have increasingly addressed controlled interventions to reduce distress. Medical outcome is also being tested in several recent studies. (See excellent review by Levenson and Bemis (1991) for a critical assessment of research studies.)[23] Clearly, prospective controlled studies using appropriate sampling methods and quantitative instruments are resulting in data that offer far more reliability and hence, scientific validity.

The explosion of mind-body research in cancer has great appeal to the public and to alternative and complementary cancer therapy practitioners. While the visibility of recent studies by Spiegel and colleagues (1989)[27] and Fawzy and colleagues (1990)[6,7] have brought visibility to the field, expectations have also been enhanced. The overinterpretation of early results is tempting in the search for rapid answers to difficult questions for which patients urgently seek. Because of increasing information and the potential for misuse of data in these areas, it is important that mental health professionals and chaplains working in cancer have a firm knowledge base from which to advise patients, their families and colleagues in oncology. This review provides an update on information in the areas outlined below:

A. Current status of clinical research;
B. New stresses on healthy individuals with enhanced cancer risk;
C. New stresses on patients and families;
D. Guidelines for clinicians.

Current Status of Clinical Research

The advances in psychological assessment research have occurred concurrent with advances in endocrinology, and more recently immunology. These events have spawned an identified research area which explores brain, endocrine and immune function and how they may impact upon cancer morbidity and mortality: psychoneuroimmunology. This research spans the range of psychophysiological responses that may impact on tumor growth. For example, a study by Bovbjerg, Redd and colleagues (1990) suggests the immune system "learns" from repeated exposures to an immunosuppressive agent, so that immunosuppression occurs *before* the drug is given. Similar to the conditioned nausea and vomiting which develops after several cycles of cancer chemotherapy.[2]

The result of the diverse research areas which explore psychosocial and behavioral factors in cancer has led to collaboration of individuals with backgrounds that are widely different. This allows for hybridization of ideas and stimulation to develop novel approaches to research. However, it also leads to slower assimilation and collaboration of investigators and difficulty in identifying funding resources. Two major research domains have evolved: one, constituting primarily cancer control and epidemiological research; and, the other, the psychological, social, psychiatric and psychoneuroimmune domain. Behavioral research contributes to both domains:

Prevention research		Psychological
Cancer control	Behavioral	Social
Epidemiology		Psychiatric
		Psychoneuroimmune

While there are many gains from this broad base of research, there are also difficulties because it is not a unitary area of oncologic research with identified researchers.

For purposes of this update on psychosocial and behavioral research in cancer, studies are reviewed and critiqued in five areas:

a. Life style and behaviors
b. Social environment
c. Personality and coping
d. Affective states/life events
e. Psychosocial/behavioral interventions
f. Spiritual/existential

Each of the five areas is discussed and summarized by providing an estimate of the likely contribution to cancer morbidity and mortality, taking available studies into account. Judgment for inclusion as a positive factor in morbidity/mortality is based on presence of one or more positive studies and absence of significant conflicting negative studies. The list is not inclusive and the judgment made is a personal opinion. The reader is referred to more extensive reviews available.[1,21]

a. Life Style and Behaviors

The most clear findings of a relationship between cancer and behavior through exposure to carcinogenic substances and life style habits exist in this area.[14] Changing habits in the U.S. appear to parallel increasing public education efforts about the health hazards of smoking and increasing pressure on the tobacco industry to attack the leading exposure which increases cancer risk. Alcohol, while a major co-factor in oropharyngeal cancer, receives far less in the way of public education concerning its cancer risk. Diet is becoming far more healthful as individuals who are health-conscious reduce fat, increase fiber in their diet and avoid obesity, recognizing their relationship to cancer. Sexual habits in relation to AIDS, are moving to greater use of protection. Information about viral origin of cervical cancer and women's sexual exposure history needs more public awareness. Habits have changed about sun bathing and tanning in new melanoma prevention efforts. In addition, studies to understand delay and factors which contribute to later stage cancer at time of diagnosis continue.

In summary:

Behavior	Morbidity	Mortality
Tobacco Use	Yes	Yes
Alcohol	Yes	Yes
Diet (Fat, fiber)	Yes	Yes
Sun Exposure	Yes	Yes
Sexual Exposures	Yes	Yes
Delay Behavior	Yes	Yes

b. Social Environment

The effect of individuals' social environment is increasingly identified as having a contribution to cancer morbidity and mortality.[9,10] Individuals who are economically disadvantaged suffer from poor access to health care, but in addition, factors such as nutritional deficiencies, greater presence of other medical illnesses, crowding and chronic stress of poverty are factors that have not been well studied for their relative separate contribution. A recent study by Cella[5] and colleagues of 2400 patients treated by standardized protocols in a clinical trial group found that education and income correlated with shorter survival, when controlled for known predictors of outcome.

Data from a meta analysis of six studies has shown that poor or absent social ties have an impact on overall morbidity and mortality from a range of diseases, including cancer.[16] A study by Levy and colleagues[22] suggests an impact of social support on NK activity in women with breast cancer.

Estimates in regard to social environment suggest:

	Morbidity	Mortality
Low socioeconomic status[6,14]	Yes	Yes
Low education[6]		Yes
Poor, absent ties[16]	Yes	Yes
Alone vs. married[9]		Yes

c. Personality, Traits and Coping Styles

It is in this area that data are most difficult to critique because different studies present directly conflicting conclusions, making an overall estimate difficult. Type C personality has been studied by Temoshock in an attempt to examine the effect of poor emotional expression on outcome. Her studies of melanoma are provocative but are not yet replicated.[29] Type A personality was examined by Fox in an analysis of the Western Collaborative cardiovascular sample.[8] The relative risk of type A (with repeated arousal) reached 1.5 Relative Risk, due to greater smoking history. Fighting spirit, studied by Greer and colleagues[11] offered an interesting survival advantage; however, several studies of breast cancer and other sites have proven negative for such predictors.[4a,18,14a] A study by Holland and colleagues[14] of women's survival from Stage II breast cancer at eight years showed no survival advantage for any subscale of the SCL-90 at time of beginning chemotherapy. The finding of anger as a positive predictor by Derogatis has not been confirmed and Cella noted the levels of distress on which differences were based largely less than a standard deviation and illness severity may have differed. Nevertheless, the proposed areas are as follows:

	Morbidity	*Mortality*
Type C[29]	?	?
Type A[8]	-	- (1.5RR)
Fighting spirit[11,4a,18,14a]	No	?
Anger	-	No
Negative studies[18,4a,14]	Yes	Yes

d. Affective States and Life Events

Bereavement and depression have been most extensively studied for a role in cancer morbidity and mortality. They have also been most carefully examined for immune correlates in physically healthy individuals. In terms of bereavement, the more carefully bereavement studies have been controlled the more they have failed to confirm a relationship to cancer onset or mortality.[13] Depression, likewise, despite early positive studies[24] has shown less correlation with increased cancer morbidity or mortality in later studies.[3,12,19] The large prospective study by Zonderman and colleagues of a nationally representative sample is the most recent persuasive evidence showing that individuals who had depressive symptoms or depression did not die of cancer in the following 10 years than did individuals who had not been depressed 10 years earlier.[32] The fact that immune changes have accompanied depressive and grieving symptoms has been of great interest for potential clinical effects.[17] One study showed a protective effect for social support.[1a] However, a review by Stein and co-workers has raised questions about interpretation of psychoimmune data in relation to depressive symptoms.[28]

Chronic distress as representative of psychiatric disorders did not predict cancer mortality.[20] Anxiety has not been studied and may be increasingly important as we see individuals living with knowledge of enhanced genetic cancer risk who have chronic anxiety. A recent study by Ramirez suggests stressful events were related to breast cancer relapse.[26] A symbolically meaningful occasion, in a well designed study of a Chinese holiday honored by older women, resulted in briefly postponed death from disease including cancer, which was followed after the holiday by a peak in deaths.[25] This observation raises interesting opportunities for speculation about the mechanism.

	Morbidity	Immune	Mortality
Bereavement[13]	No	Mild	No
Bereavement/Social Support[1a]	-	Immuno competence	-
Depression/Symptoms 3,12,17,19,24,28,32	No	Mild	No
Neuroticism/Distress[20]	No	Unk	No
Anxiety (healthy individuals)	Unk	Mild	Unk
Stressful events[10,26,8a]	?	Mild	Relapse
Symbolic occasions[25]	-	-	(Briefly postponed)

e. Psychosocial Interventions

The findings from many studies identifying nature and frequency of distress in cancer patients have led to increasing intervention studies with attempts at improving coping and well being. Over 20 studies, using a range of interventions, have showed enhanced well being. A positive effect on outcome of cancer has only been reported by Spiegel and colleagues (1989).[27] Fawzy and co-workers showed a positive effect of intervention on immune function in Stage I and II melanoma.[6,7] Psychotropic drug studies have also enhanced quality of life. However, three studies, two of them recent, have found holistic efforts carried out by alternative therapy approaches did not have an effect on mortality.[4,23,1] *but on quality of life.*

Morbidity		QL	Immune	Mortality
Psychosocial/Behavior				
Interventions (>20 studies)	-	Yes	Unk	No
Spiegel et al. 1989[27]	-	Yes	Unk	Yes
Fawzy et al. 1990[28]	-	Yes	Yes	Unk
Alternative therapies[4,1,23]	-	Yes	Unk	No

f. Spiritual/Existential

An area of coping with serious illness which has been neglected by social scientists is that of the degree to which individuals rely on spiritual and religious beliefs in coping with an illness. Several studies have shown that such beliefs lead to enhanced coping and greater life satisfaction.[33] There is a new effort to include use of religion and belief systems in models of stress and coping (Figure 1). They impact positively upon maintaining hope, reducing distress and retaining a sense of control over events. These intrinsic beliefs, including belief in a higher power to whom prayers can be directed, are coupled with the comfort derived from participation in religious rituals and the availability of a community of individuals that provides social and concrete support and help during illness. A current study of patients at Memorial and at the Hadassah Medical Center in Jerusalem will test the impact of each aspect on coping.

New Stresses on Healthy Individuals

The explosion of information in the field of molecular genetics has resulted in new cancer information being given to the public: the knowledge of genetic risk of a particular type of cancer. Women today recognize enhanced breast cancer risk when a first degree relative develops it. Colon cancer, and more recently ovarian cancer, are becoming known by the public to have a genetic contribution. Early detection becomes critically important for these individu-

FIGURE 1. (Adapted from Kobasa, 1982)

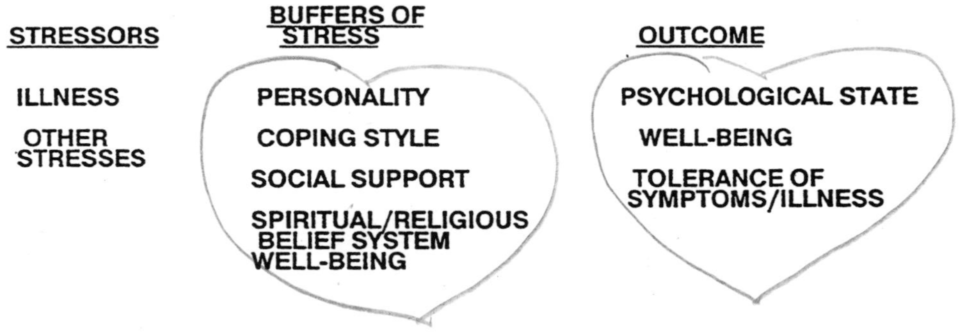

STRESSORS

ILLNESS

OTHER
STRESSES

BUFFERS OF
STRESS

PERSONALITY

COPING STYLE

SOCIAL SUPPORT

SPIRITUAL/RELIGIOUS
BELIEF SYSTEM
WELL-BEING

OUTCOME

PSYCHOLOGICAL STATE

WELL-BEING

TOLERANCE OF
SYMPTOMS/ILLNESS

als, and therefore participation in screening is essential. However, in some syndromes, such as Li-Fraumeni, knowledge of risk at an early age cannot be accompanied by a behavior to reduce risk or even detection. The result is a new population of "worried well" who have chronic anxiety. Kash and Holland have demonstrated the effect of such knowledge of high risk on women's detection surveillance behavior, for breast cancer which is an example of a new psychological issue confronting the public about cancer.

In addition, far more information is available about factors which may *reduce* cancer risk. Healthy individuals now question whether to participate in clinical trials, in which as tamoxifen and other chemo preventive substances are used to reduce cancer risk. Individuals with morbid fears of cancer become excessively concerned about these issues.

New Stresses on Patients and Families

The impact of the mind-body research, particularly the intervention studies, has focused attention on the need for improved psychological support of patients. Watson (1991) has edited an excellent review of psychosocial interventions in cancer.[31] Mind-body research, however, has encouraged expectation that positive emotions and psychosocial interventions alter cancer outcome. Approaches such as the Exceptional Cancer Patients (ECP) carry with them the counter belief that attitudes may have caused the tumor and negative attitudes may enhance tumor growth. Gray and Doan (1990) have offered a helpful sociological perspective.[9a] Cancer is a frightening disease that elicits in some patients the need to become a mythic "heroic warrior" who bravely "fights cancer," as suggested by some programs as ECP. Coping in any other style causes the patient to feel guilty and inadequate. The concerned relative may feel the patient is "allowing the tumor to grow."

Those who are distressed or unable to use it should be reminded that three controlled studies of holistic and mind-body interventions did not show any survival advantage for those who participated as compared to those who received conventional care alone.[4,1,23]

The other major new stressor for patients is the change in the patient role in decision making. The new participation as a partner

in care is helpful and constructive. However, the present day cus-
tom too often does not take into account the patients' needs and
responses. Physicians, fearful of legal repercussions, sometimes
leave the decision to the patient, after offering highly different op-
tions for treatment. Anxiety, fearfulness, and worries of making
"the wrong decision" plague many patients and their families. The
pendulum needed to swing to permit greater patient participation,
but it needs to swing back toward the center.

Guidelines for Clinicians

It is important to keep up-to-date on the rapidly growing body of
psychosocial and behavioral research. Clinical investigations are
turning now to more controlled trials of interventions which will
soon provide more clear guidelines for clinicians for offering psychological support and assistance in coping. In addition, a clinician
must also know the popular holistic and complementary cancer
therapies in order to be able to advise colleagues, patients and families.[30] One should support those interventions that are helpful to
patients, explaining how and why they may be. The people should
be encouraged to return if they feel distressed by the intervention,
and discouraged not to try those that may be physically deleterious
or psychologically distressing.

Guidelines for patients which can be safely applied, based on the
clinical and research data available, in regard to psychosocial and
behavioral factors, are the following:

1. Use the American Cancer Society guidelines for early detection of cancer (Pap smear, mammogram); avoid sun exposure;
   diet advice (high fiber, vegetables, low fat); avoid obesity.
2. Do not assume cancer equals death. Early cancer is curable.
3. Become a partner with the physician in your care.
4. Do not keep your worries about illness a secret from those
   who love you. Support helps.
5. Do not believe you brought cancer on yourself.
6. Do not feel guilty if you aren't thinking "positively" all the
   time.

7. Use ways of coping that have worked for you in the past. Don't feel you must "fight cancer" in a particular model; just because the model works for someone else does not mean it is "the only way" or right for you.
8. Consider exploring value systems and spiritual beliefs that helped before; social and religious communities which share your beliefs are often available to help you.
9. Use support and self help groups that make you feel better; leave any that make you feel worse.
10. Use mind-body methods that help you cope; disregard unhelpful aspects.
11. Nutritional and chemical alternative treatments should be checked with your physician; never stop traditional treatment in favor of a complementary or alternative therapy.

REFERENCES

1. Bagenal, F.S., Easton, D.F., Harris, E. et al. (1990). Survival of patients with breast cancer attending Bristol Cancer Help Centre. *The Lancet* 336: 606-610.

1a. Baron, R.S., Cutrona, C.E., Hecklin, D. et al. (1990). Social support and immune function among spouses of cancer patients. *J. Personality and Social Psych.* 59:344-352.

2. Bovbjerg, D.H., Redd, W.H., Maier, L.A., Holland, J.C., Lesko, L.M., Niedzwiecki, D. and Rubin, S.C., Hakes, T.B. (1990). Anticipatory immune suppression and nausea in women receiving cyclic chemotherapy for ovarian cancer. *J Consult Clin Psych* 58:153-157.

3. Bielauskas, L.A., Garron, D.C. (1982). Psychological depression and cancer. *Gen. Hosp. Psychiatry* 4:187-195.

4. Cassileth, B.R., Lusk, E.J., Guerry, D., Blake, A.D., Walsh, W.P., Kascius, L., Schultz, D.J. (1991). Survival and quality of life among patients receiving unproven as compared with conventional cancer therapy. *New Eng J of Med* 324:1180-1185.

4a. Cassileth, B.R., Lusk, E.J., Miller, D.J. et al. (1985): Psychological correlates of survival in advanced malignant disease? *New Eng J of Med* 312: 1551-1555.

5. Cella, D.F., Orav, J,, Kornblith, A.B., Holland, J.C. et al. (1991). Socioeconomic status and cancer survival. *J of Clin Oncology* 9:1500-1509.

6. Fawzy, F.I., Cousins, N., Fawzy, W.W. et al. (1990). A structured psychiatric intervention for cancer patients, I: Changes over time in methods of coping and affective disturbance. *Arch Gen Psychiatry* 47:720-725.

7. Fawzy, F.I., Kemeny, M.E., Fawzy, W. et al. (1990). A structured psychiatric intervention for cancer patients, II: Changes over time in immunologic measures. *Arch Gen Psychiatry* 47:729-735.

8. Fox, B.H., Ragland, D.R., Brand, R.J., Rosenman, R.H. (1987). Type A behavior and cancer mortality. *Ann NY Acad of Sciences* 496:620-627.

8a. Goodkin, K., Antoni, M.H., Blarney, P.H. (1986): Stress and hopelessness in the promotion of cervical cancer. *J Psychosom Res* 39:67-76.

9. Goodwin, J.S., Hunt, W.C., Key, C.R., Samet, J.M. (1987). The effect of marital status on stage of treatment and survival of cancer patients. *New Eng J of Med* 258: 3125-3130.

9a. Gray, R.E. and Doan, B.D. (1990). Heroic self-healing and cancer: clinical issues for the health profession. *J of Palliative Care* 6:32-41.

10. Graham, S., Snell, L.M., Graham, J.B. et al. (1971) Social trauma in the epidemiology of cancer of the cervix. *J. Chronic Dis* 24:711-735.

11. Greef, S., Morris, T., Pettingale, K.W. (1979). Psychological response to breast cancer; effect on outcome. *Lancet* 2:785-787.

12. Hahn, R.C., Petitti, D.B. (1988). Minnesota Multiphasic Personality Inventory-rated depression and the incidence of breast cancer. *Cancer* 61:845-848.

13. Helsing, K.J., Szklo, M. (1981). Mortality after bereavement. *Am J Epidemiol* 1124:41-52.

14. Holland, J.C. (1989). Behavioral and psychosocial risk factors in cancer: human studies. In: J.C. Holland and J.H. Rowland (Eds.), *Handbook of Psycho-oncology*. Oxford University Press, New York, 705-726.

14a. Holland, J.C., Korzun, A.H., Tross, S., Cella, D.F. et al. (1986). Psychosocial factors and disease-free survival in Stage II breast cancer. (Abstract) *Proc Am Soc Clin Oncol* 5.237.

15. Holland, J.C. (1989). Fears and abnormal reactions to cancer in physically Healthy Individuals. In J.C. Holland and J.H. Rowland (Eds.) *Handbook of Psychooncology*. Oxford University Press, New York 13-21.

16. House, J.S., Landis, K.R., Umberson, D. (1988). Social relationships and health. *Science* 240:540-545.

17. Irwin, M., Daniels, M., Weiner, H. (1987). Immune and neuroendocrine changes during bereavement. *Psychiatr Clin North Am* 10:449-465.

18. Jamison, R.N., Burish, T.G., Wallston, K.A. (1987). Psychogenic factors in predicting survival of breast cancer patients. *J Clin Oncol* 5:768-772.

19. Kaplan, G.A., Reynolds, P. (1988). Depression and cancer mortality and morbidity: prospective evidence from the Alameda county study. *J Behav Med* 11:1-13.

20. Kash K. M., Holland, J.C., Halper, M. S. et al. (1992). Psychological distress and surveillance behaviors of women with a family history of breast cancer. *J Natl Cancer Institute* 84: 24-30.

21. Keehn, R.J. (1980). Follow-up studies of World War II and Korean conflict prisoners. *Am J Epidemiol* 111:194-211.

22. Levenson, J.C. and Bemis, C. (1991). The Role of Psychological Factors in Cancer Onset and Progression. *Psychosomatics* 32:125-132.

23. Levy, S.M., Herberman, R.B., Whiteside, T. et al. (1990). Perceived social support and tukmor estrogen /progesterone receptoro status as predictors of natural killer cell activity in breast cancer patients. *Psychosom Med* 52:73-85.

24. Morganstein, H., Gellert, G.H., Walter, S.D. et al. (1984). The impact of a psychosocial support program on survival with breast cancer; the importance of selection bias in program evaluation. *J of Chron Diseases* 37:273-282.

25. Persky, V.W., Kempthorne-Rawson, J., Shekelle, R.P. (1987): Personality and risk of cancer: 20-year follow-up of the Western Electric Study. *Psychosom Med* 49:435-449.

26. Phillips, D.P. and Smith, D.G. (1990). Postponement of Death Until Symbolically Meaningful Occasions. *JAMA* 263: 1947-1951.

27. Ramirez, A.J., Craig, T.K., Watson, J.P. et al. (1989). Stress and relapse of breast cancer. Br Med J 298:291-293.

28. Spiegel, P., Bloom, J.R., Kraemer, H.C. et al. (1989). Effects of psychosocial treatment on survival of patients with metastatic breast cancer. *Lancet* 2:888-892.

29. Stein, M., Miller, A.H., and Trestman, R.L. (1991). Depression of the Immune System and Health and Illness. *Arch Gen Psych* 48:171-177.

30. Temoshok, L., Heller, B.W., Sageviel, R.W. et al. (1985). The relationship of psychological factors of prognostic indicators in cutaneous malignant melanoma. *J Psychosom Res* 29:139-153.

31. U.S. Congress, office of Technology Assessment, 1990. Unconventional cancer treatments (OTA-H-405). Wash DC: U.S. Govt Printing Office.

32. Watson, M. (Ed.) (1991). *Cancer Patient Care: Psychosocial Treatment Methods.* Cambridge University Press, Cambridge, U.K.

33. Zonderman, A.B., Costa, P.T., Jr., McCrae, R.R. (1989). Depression as a risk for cancer morbidity and mortality in a nationally representative sample. *JAMA* 262:1191-1195.

34. Yates, J.W. et al. (1981). Religion in patients with advanced cancer. *Med Pediatr Oncol*, 9:121-128.

Counselor of Quality

Avery D. Weisman, MD

How best to cope with cancer is both a practical challenge and a metaphor for joining religion and medicine. Their combined purpose in this respect is to help patients and other concerned individuals cope with what seems an unreasonable burden at times, as well as to preserve a passable quality of life while undergoing treatment and its aftermath. I shall discuss what I consider relevant issues under four major headings:

1. Safe conduct
2. Coping
3. Social support
4. Counselors of quality.

SAFE CONDUCT

Safe conduct is the care we offer patients and significant others, in addition to medical treatment and physical care. It combines external factors, such as living arrangements that help maintain quality of life, hospice care, strengthening family ties, financial resources, and so on, with internal factors such as strengths shared with others. Consequently, *safe conduct* is a combination of *morale*, which is confidence in the ability to cope, and *quality of life*, which means all the external factors that encourage an ill individual to retain a sense of satisfaction, sustenance, and purpose.

What is safe conduct? It is an offer of safety, security, sustenance, and self-esteem—a rather lofty obligation—but it helps keep expectation and demand within realistic limits. It means guiding someone safely where there is no assurance of safety; it means offering security under very intimidating circumstances; it means establishing an alliance, despite the solitude of suffering and bereavement. Safe conduct is trying to make the most of being alive and alert to the reality beyond the sickbed. It is coping with pressure points of the practical problems of living and dying. It is the here-and-now of anticipatory bereavement.

The counselor needs safe conduct, too; otherwise, the outcome is burnout, which is a result of being fatigued, unappreciated, resentful, too ambitious or desperate, or feeling that efforts are inconsequential. Caregivers can experience demoralization as well as depression, anxiety, or other forms of distress.

COPING

Coping may be defined as what we do about a problem, once it has been identified. It has, therefore, two parts: (1) assessing what is wrong, and (2) acting upon and maybe correcting a problem to bring about some relief, if not total resolution.

There are many ways to cope, and some strategies work better than others. Strategies that prepare and evaluate potential consequences are apt to work better than strategies that passively wait and see. Good copers tend, in general, to be assertive, not angry or doing something for its own sake, but feeling they have something to say about how leading problems are to be resolved.

Problems are always in great supply and are recognized by their association with (1) *anxiety,* which means worry about a precarious future; (2) *ambiguity,* which involves confusion about what some predicament means; and (3) *ambivalence,* which concerns itself with uncertain relationships and acceptance or repudiation of potential social support.

Coping well with *anxiety* should lead to relief of distress and return to comparative equilibrium. The goal of coping is composure without emotional extremes.

Coping well with *ambiguity* should correct doubt and confusion about what is going on and clarify the meaning of threatening events.

Coping well with *ambivalence* should settle indecision and reluctance about accepting support from others who want to be supportive.

The opposite of coping well is increased vulnerability or a disposition to become distressed.

I do not expect that a more or less abstract discussion about coping will be very effective. Actually, it is more important to consider the qualities of good copers; because only by emulating those who do cope well, do we learn to use our knowledge and compassion and become counselors of quality.

Good copers are generally flexible, resourceful, pragmatic, and optimistic. I don't mean that they are always ready to go, never tired, seldom discouraged, and "full of pep." Because coping with cancer requires so much, hardly anyone would be justified in trying to be this offensive caricature of a caregiver.

Caregivers who are optimists do not always cope well: they may misjudge the handicaps and expect too much. Pessimists, however, will probably fail too often by giving up and resorting to strategies that deal with other kinds of problems besides helping the patient. The key idea about optimism and pessimism is that optimists believe in themselves and their capacity, while pessimists are ruled unnecessarily by much self-doubt. Counselling cancer patients requires skill and reasonable willingness to accept small gains. Good copers cannot be extremists in any regard. They keep cool, but concerned and composed under most circumstances. Flexibility means that they have a reserve to call upon without being committed to only one or two methods of approaching patients. Goals are within reach and, therefore, efforts are more likely to be helpful and hopeful. Regardless of the circumstances, good copers usually can manage a little gain or benefit, believing in their own values and standards, because this is that they judge themselves by.

SOCIAL SUPPORT

"Being supportive" is an empty phrase. It tells very little about what a counselor will or should be doing under what circumstances. Support ranges from providing tangible assistance in money, food, and shelter, to much longer efforts to guide, direct, inform, interpret, and so on. In other words, the term, "social support," covers even psychotherapy and much counseling, however brief and problem-centered.

I see the meaning of social support in the following way: it is to bring about *normalization* and *acceptability* of the client/patient by various interventions. It does not mean vague or hit-and-miss use of open encouragement, facile phrases, and so on. It is always substantial and backed up by an understanding of what is wrong and what must either be eliminated or supported. Social support does not promise exact goals or permanent change; it does tend to foster some type of corrective action that normalizes and makes behavior more acceptable. It is meant to be short-term and is best when the patient/client feels empowered to utilize his/her social support networks. The true meaning of social support is doing something to improve *morale*, that quiet sense of confidence in one's own capacity that permits regular confrontation with difficulties.

COUNSELORS OF QUALITY

What does a counselor with a religious or pastoral bent have to offer cancer patients that other kinds of counselors do not? What are the strengths and resources that are more or less special to the pastoral orientation?

In the first place, I believe that a pastoral counselor has an *acceptability* to many patients that a psychologist, social worker, and certainly a psychiatrist does not. It is *normal* to talk with a pastoral counselor–however tactful and diplomatic the types of counselors may be, there is always a tinge of sickness and aberration that qualifies negatively whatever kind of relationship may result.

In the second place, cancer patients at any stage or phase, are vulnerable not merely to disease and the complications of illness and its treatment, but to questions that may be called *ultimate questions*, that have no sure answers except what an individual stands for and is responsible to. This is the *suprapersonal dimension*, which considers and takes very seriously problems of individuality in its relation to the totality of whatever there is or might be. It is not meant to be preachy at all, but it does draw upon the best in counselors of quality.

Counselors of quality have an established social identity. This is credibility too, because it matches up to expectation and even fits in with what the leading problems require and need for resolution.

A counselor of quality, therefore, has four main qualities, virtues, or talents. These are *character*, *credentials*, *credibility*, and *compassion*. Define them in any way you wish, but remember that each trait or talent works with the others and fails to work without an assist from the others.

Any counselor needs to be aware of his/her inner strengths and resources in order to cope with personal vulnerability and thus learn from fallibility. Part of a counselor's job is not only to recognize strengths, shortcomings, and problems in patient/clients, but to identify points where *denial* is the only strategy at work. Counselors must be able to confront incipient bereavement without denial, yet with much social support. It takes courage, morale, and of course credibility and belief in the capacity to cope.

PRACTICAL SUMMARY

Coping with cancer from the patient's or the counselor's viewpoint means that strengths and resources depend on assessing predominant problems and acting appropriately to alleviate them. It does not always mean resolution of problems, but it does require understanding where the pressure points are that lead to more distress. Thus, counselors anticipate as well as understand actual distress; visualize various outcomes of different interventions, medical or otherwise; and narrow the gap between what is hoped for and what might be possible.

Pastoral counseling needs a viewpoint that maintains morale in the utmost phase of terminal illness. Facing mortality is difficult for the counselor as well as significant others. Therefore, they must deal directly with bereavement and potential loss, if possible, indicating their willingness to confront ultimate questions, even without answers. Overall, the purpose of quality counseling is in the counselor: limitation is not futility. The job of counselling is not to figure out the universe or explain the unexplainable. Rather, the purpose of counseling is to help a suffering individual to come back within the range of normalized behavior and to become acceptable and credible. In this way, out of the web of vulnerability can come further strengths and resources.

Where Do Chaplains Fit in the World of Cancer Care?

George Handzo, MDiv

Where do we as chaplains fit in the world of cancer care? How do religious professionals respond to people who have this disease, are trying to cope with it, and have beliefs about it?

I am convinced that we have to approach what we *do* by being clear about who we *are*. First, we are explicitly and publicly people of religious faith. Obviously, many other health care professionals are also people of faith. However, we alone advertise that belief on our name tags. Our title says at least as much about our religious views as it does about our credentials. Patients, family members or staff might disagree or be confused about what we are supposed to *do*. However, I suspect that every one of them would suppose that chaplains are people who believe in a god and that that belief is important, even central, in their lives.

Second, we represent a religious community. To be a certified chaplain or congregational clergyperson, we must be ordained, consecrated, endorsed or otherwise set aside by *some* particular religious group. Unlike any other health care profession, our titles do not simply certify that we have a particular set of skills and credentials. They also certify that we are authorized and even expected to represent the views of a group that is probably not even our employer. The hospital only gives us permission to function and maybe gives us the resources. Our *authority* comes from our religious community.

Unfortunately, we have sometimes regarded these realities as a liability rather than as a strength. We have wanted to counteract the old image of the chaplain as the simplistic preacher who was ignorant of medical and psychological issues and unable to operate within the hospital system. We have wanted to become full-fledged members of the health care team. To attain this admirable goal, we have had to learn the customs and language of science. We have adopted psychological theory and practice. For the most part, we have been successful in defining a new role and a new image for ourselves. Chaplains are more integrated into the health care team than ever before. We know we belong. We are capable of matching credentials, jargon, and quality assurance plans with anyone in our institutions.

However, along the way, we may have swung the pendulum too far and lost part of our heritage. While trying to bridge science and religion, we have instead helped perpetuate the myth that they cannot coexist by assuming that we have to speak *either* the language of psychology or the language of religion rather than a combination of the two. We have often been embarrassed by God talk. To be sure, we still use it in our own groups and behind the curtains in patient rooms. But we have been reticent to acknowledge to other health care professionals that we are, basically, believers in God. As we have gone on in this way, we have lost some of our ability to speak theologically. We have pretended that we can counsel in a style that excludes our values and beliefs from the interaction.

Being people of faith and representatives of a religious community *must* color what we do. That coloring is certainly clear to those with whom we work. It must be at least that clear to us.

The basic stance of modern chaplaincy has been widely discussed so I will only touch on it here. Our intent is to be with the patients or family members where they are, to be a non-judgmental presence which affirms their worth as human beings, and to let patients lead us in the directions that are most useful for them. We walk with and support patients in the valley of the shadow of death. We help them to share or vent feelings. However, we are certainly more than friendly visitors. First, we actively pursue our task of being with rather than passively waiting for patients to decide to talk. While we try not to push patients, we definitely encourage them and let them know clearly that we are willing to listen. Second, the motivation behind what we do is clear. We value persons and have high regard for their worth because they are so regarded by the God in whom we believe.

Certainly, the willingness and ability to simply be with patients and the freedom to visit them without an agenda or a task to perform is a great gift to patients and family members. It takes great skill to build the trusting relationships that allow for this intimate sharing to occur.

However, the role outlined above can be, and is, filled by others such as well trained volunteers, nurses and social workers. Moreover, the current cost conscious atmosphere in health care is forcing us to justify our existence in ways that were never required of us before. This still evolving pressure can be a positive development. It is forcing chaplaincy as a discipline to articulate and, heaven forbid, even to quantify not only how we are necessary to good health care but how we are unique among health care professions. It is forcing us to take seriously what makes us different from other care givers rather than attempting to show that we are worthy of inclusion on the health care team because we can do anything other psychosocial professionals can do.

What is this uniqueness? Unlike any other health care profession, we are sensitive to and skilled in the discussion of spiritual and existential issues. These are issues that are not definable in the specifics of scientific language. These issues include the nature of human worthiness, what it means to exist, the realization of one's mortality, and questions of the meaning of life. They are typified by the patient who cries, "Why me?" and is not interested in a discussion of oncogenes, but in trying to speak about the unspeakable fear of worthlessness, meaninglessness, and the encounter with mortality. These issues can only be discussed in the language of story, poem, and ritual. In other words, they can only be discussed in the language that is natural to religious expression.

On some level, these issues are present for all cancer patients. As Susan Sontag has described so well, the place of cancer in our culture and the nature of the disease itself are powerful forces which invariably bring anyone who is in contact with the illness face to face with ultimate existential or spiritual concerns (Sontag, 1977).

To come to terms with a diagnosis of cancer is to restore a sense of normalcy and equilibrium to one's life. Restoring this equilibrium includes integrating the reality of cancer and its possible consequences into one's view of how the world works, how a divine power functions and what meaning and worth there is in life when one is seriously ill. If one's faith system can integrate such a challenge into its normal way of looking at the world, coping is improved.

The mother of a young pediatric patient from a fundamentalist Protestant background insisted all through treatment that her son would be healed. When it became clear that the child would die, the staff worried about how the mother would cope. Mother calmly announced to the chaplain that the problem was not with God but with her misreading of God's will for her son. Clearly, God did not will her son to live. However, since everything God does is good, some greater good must be coming from her son's death. Her job was to trust God's will and know that it was for the best.

How do we as chaplains uniquely address these issues? We have certainly gained a great deal of clinical skill from psychology. These skills, however, are not ends in themselves. They turn out to be vehicles for interpreting and tools for delivering the same messages we have wanted to transmit all along. They allow us to make our messages heard in ways we were not able to make them heard previously. My basic thesis for the rest of this chapter is that we do not so much need to invent new ways of serving patients and family members as we need to develop more sophisticated understandings of the old ways so that we can use them more efficiently and effectively.

WORSHIP

Group worship is probably the best example of one of these old ways that needs to be reinterpreted. Conducting worship is obviously one of the most traditional tasks of chaplaincy. However, in many hospitals, it has been abandoned because it took a lot of the chaplain's time and few patients came. At my institution, attendance has also dropped as the patients have become sicker and the average stay declined. However, we continue to have Jewish, Protestant, and Roman Catholic worship every weekend and on all major religious holidays. Patients and family are personally invited to every appropriate service and are escorted if necessary.

It is a lot of work. It continues to happen for several reasons. First, we have a very supportive administration and a Department of Volunteer Resources which is committed to providing us with the people to continue this program. Second, we believe that worship services provide a number of concrete benefits to patients and family members dealing with cancer. For many, it is a connection to something familiar and normal in their outside community which is clearly important in their coping with cancer. Worship can also provide an opportunity for a return to a religious community long abandoned. It is not uncommon for patients who have not attended religious services for many years to attend while in the hospital. Here, where no one knows them, they can try out this community again without embarrassment or guilt.

Worship provides a concrete tie to God. In a setting where religion can seem so foreign, worship is the best way to let people know that God is with them. It is the setting in which God has the best chance of being heard by us. I often tell students preparing to lead worship for the first time that this is their opportunity to say the things to their patients about how God works that they would have liked to have said at the bedside but did not have the proper opportunity. Worship gives us a chance to tell patients things in a group that would be too confrontive if we told them one to one.

Much has been said and written about the usefulness of support groups in helping people cope with cancer. Properly structured in an informal dialogical format, worship in the hospital is a support group. Certainly in a setting like Memorial Hospital where everyone has the same basic disease, worship allows patients and family members to share and gain support from other believers who also have cancer. Worship bears the same relationship to a private visit from a chaplain as a cancer support group bears to a private visit from a psychologist or a social worker. Finally, this support group analogy holds, not only for those who attend worship, but also for those who do not. We hear repeatedly from patients how important it was for them to have been invited to worship even though they did not attend. They felt included in the group and derived benefits simply because they were invited.

PRAYER AND RITUAL

Related to the use of worship is the use of prayer and ritual. Again, ritual is a concrete tie to a person's tradition, community, and God. It is not uncommon for patients to discover meaning in the rituals of their tradition that they never knew they had. Mrs. K., whose son was recently diagnosed with a bone tumor, asked me if I would have a Catholic priest come and bless some objects she had. She had listed herself as a Methodist. She explained that when she married she had left the Catholic Church with no regrets because the ceremonies and rituals never had had any meaning for her. She still did not understand what their meaning was for her, but she had become certain that "there is something there." We see Catholic patients who have not been to confession in decades and who previously felt that this rite had no effect on their relationship to God. These patients suddenly see confession as essential for reconciling themselves to God. Likewise, we see Jewish patients who never considered themselves observant who now want to use the resources of their tradition. We are often far too reticent as chaplains and other health care professionals to offer these religious resources to patients. We often prefer to wait for the patient who is feeling ill and out of control to suddenly seize control of the situation and ask us to do what we should do, or at least, offer without a request.

The same is true of prayer. Anyone with any experience as a chaplain has prayed with a patient who, at best, seemed cool to the idea but who wound up deeply affected by it. We often forget how powerfully prayer can tap into something deep within the patient that we cannot and do not need to understand. Certainly, prayer should not be pushed on a patient indiscriminately. However, since patients know we are people of faith, they may expect us to pray, or, certainly will not be surprised when we offer. The emphasis should not be on finding something to replace prayer so that we do not offend people when we offer. The emphasis should be on using our clinical expertise to offer prayer and ritual in a way that will maximize the patient and family member's ability to employ these powerful tools in coping with cancer.

THEOLOGICAL TALK

The natural lead in to the use of prayer and ritual with a patient is a discussion of theological issues. In general, we as chaplains have been comfortable and competent in discussing a patient's *feelings* about God. We help patients vent their anger and sense of abandonment. We share their joy when they believe that God has answered their prayers or is giving them strength. We bolster their hope in God's continued support.

I do not think we have been as strong in dealing with the *content* of a patient's belief system. One cause of our reticence in dealing with patients around issues of illness and death is that we sometimes do not know what we believe ourselves. I am not advocating a return to the days when the chaplain knew the answer and was glad to lay it on the patient no matter how ready the patient was to hear it. I am talking about being confident in our hearts and minds about who God is for us so that we can deal with the patient's theological problems with less anxiety and defensiveness. We have become expert in building up and assessing a student chaplain's clinical skills. We need to become equally expert in helping chaplains build a theology. I am not saying that chaplains should have some particular set of beliefs although some belief systems clearly are more conducive to helping patients than others. However, to become a chaplain one should have come to some conclusion for oneself about certain core theological questions.

In addition to knowing what we ourselves believe, we need to know how these questions are dealt with in theological systems other than our own. In the modern model of chaplaincy, a chaplain may be assigned to a particular nursing unit to work with all patients regardless of religious affiliation. To make this model work, the chaplain must be able to deal with each patient within that patient's particular theological framework. It is therefore incumbent upon the chaplain to understand at least the outlines of that framework so he or she can maneuver comfortably within it. The task is similar to dealing with patients in a foreign language or dealing with patients who use coping mechanisms very different from our own. We need to understand the patient's coping pattern so that we can help that patient maximize its strengths and minimize its weaknesses.

In addition to the systems themselves, we need to be familiar with the resources that are useful within that system. For Jews and Christians that means at least familiarity with the Psalms. It is here that patients can find the whole range of their feelings toward God expressed more clearly. The juxtaposition of anger and praise within the same Psalm often helps to validate the patient's seemingly contradictory feelings. Additionally, Christians need to know how the healing stories of the Gospels are used by different faith groups. Again, using them effectively necessitates first coming to terms with what they mean for us. One litmus test is to ask ourselves if we have or could preach on one of these stories at a hospital worship service.

Finally, we need to be able to interpret the beliefs and rituals of patients to the staff. What does a Pentacostal patient mean when she says, "God will take care of me"? How can one construct a nursing care plan that takes into account the ritual needs of an Orthodox Jewish man? Chaplains can assist staff by helping them understand the patient's belief system so that staff may feel more comfortable dealing with questions of religious belief and practice.

ASSESSMENT

Another area in which we need to improve our practice is assessment. Assessment has long been looked down on in many chaplaincy circles because it violates the non-invasive, gives the patient control, lack of agenda stance of modern chaplaincy. Indeed, the concept of assessment does put us in a bind. We do want to preserve as much as possible the non-invasive quality of chaplaincy visits and our ability to be there simply for what the patient wants.

However, the practice of chaplaincy is not completely passive in terms of how topics are raised in a conversation. We clearly do not simply respond to what the patient brings up. We do raise questions in areas not initiated by the patient such as how they understand their illness medically and what their support systems are like. In the same way, we need to know how they understand their illness theologically. It is no longer good enough to say that we cannot bring up this topic with patients because they may feel pressured or interrogated when there are many other content areas that we routinely raise. If the difference between us and friendly visitors is our expertise in dealing with theological issues, then we need to make more effort to engage patients in this area. If we are going to help patients with these issues, we need to know what they believe.

The question is not, "should we assess?" but "how can we assess in a way that is effective but minimally intrusive?" A number of possibilities present themselves. In a long term care facility, some sort of spiritual assessment instrument could be used on admission. Many patients will give us an opening by identifying their affiliation or something about their faith in the conversation. Too often we treat comments such as, "Well, I just keep praying" or "God has been good to me" as cliches offered for the chaplain's benefit. They may be exactly that. However, they open the door for us to inquire about what belief may be behind these statements. In short, we need to heighten our awareness of the openings that patients do give us and be more aggressive in following them up. Any statement or question that has the slightest amount of religious content should be followed up on as a way to open up this area of inquiry.

What about the patient who does not give us any of these openings? This area needs a great deal more study and discussion than is possible here. A direct approach is to simply ask something like, "Is religious faith a part of how you are coping with this illness?" The challenge for all of us who are chaplains is to try to be more aggressive in this area of inquiry. We need to become more attuned to the issues that need to be assessed and learn to work them into our regular visiting styles. If we become comfortable with the idea of spiritual assessment, then the exact questions will come naturally.

THEOLOGICAL ISSUES

What are the theological issues that we ought to be concerned with? Many questions and statements commonly heard from patients are suggestive. "Why is God doing this to me?" "What did I do to deserve this?" "God will heal me." "I know God is with me no matter what." I have found it most helpful to treat all of the preceding as branches from a single trunk. For me, that trunk represents the question, "What is the nature of God's interaction with individual human beings in the world today?" This is the central issue dealt with by Rabbi Kushner in *When Bad Things Happen to Good People* (Kushner, 1981). It is the central issue he had to settle for himself in order to deal with the death of his son. I think our central task as chaplains to people with cancer is to aid them in confronting this question and formulating a response for themselves which helps them to cope with their disease.

The first part of the issue is, "Does God have the power to intervene and make a difference in people's lives?" Contrary to Rabbi Kushner's conclusion, virtually everyone I have ever met who has any use for a god at all would be clear that their God can make a difference. In fact, a large part of their dilemma is rooted in the belief that God could intervene and prevent or cure cancer if God chose to do so.

The question then becomes, "Why *doesn't* God intervene?" Most patients will come to the conclusion that the illness must have occurred because of something they did or did not do. The fact that they come to this conclusion is partly attributable to their desire for some explanation and the seeming lack of any alternative.

The other factors that lead to this self blame are the pervasiveness of low self esteem and the insistence of our culture that one is valued according to what one has achieved. I think the hardest concept for patients to accept is that God can truly love and value them without regard to what they have done or not done. I am sure we all hear routinely from patients like the young mother I recently visited who kept saying, "I can't get over the feeling that God wants something from me before he heals me?" She was also the woman who was bitterly disappointed when her second look surgery came back positive. She was totally convinced that with all the people she had praying for her, she would have no cancer left.

Dealing with patients around this issue is extremely delicate. To suggest to a patient that their god cannot or will not do anything for them leaves them abandoned. Even if one agrees with Kushner that God either is not omnipotent or is uninvolved, that conclusion is not helpful. God is then good for nothing. Patients will not and cannot be expected to want anything to do with a God who has nothing to offer them.

The patients and family members who come to the most helpful resolution of these issues are those who abandon the questions about what God "does." They come to the conclusion or intuitively understand that these questions are probably unanswerable and, even if they could be answered, the answers would not be helpful. These people take the attitude spelled out most clearly by John Claypool in his book, *Tracks of a Fellow Struggler* (Claypool, 1974). Claypool's idea is that what God may or may not "do" for us is not nearly as important as who God "is" for us. For Claypool, God is that one who does not fail to support us and be with us so that we never have to bear anything by ourselves. God becomes the helper in the little story called "Footprints." God is the one who walks next to us when things are going well and carries us in times of trouble. God does not help us avoid trouble or solve the problems for us, but is with us as a caregiver. Therefore, we do not solve the problem of what God does and why. We simply abandon the question as unhelpful.

My experience is that generally patients are most able to use God as a resource when they can focus on God the comforter rather than on God the doer. Certainly, we do not want to short circuit patients' needs to process their feelings. We do not want to rush to a solution before a patient is ready to hear it. However, we must abandon the idea that we are never directive with a patient or that we can only go where they lead us. Rather than feeling manipulated, many patients welcome suggestions about new ways of viewing God. We must understand that a theological system that is not helping the patient is a dysfunctional coping mechanism. It is our job as health care professionals to assist the patient in strengthening that coping mechanism.

SHAME AND GUILT

In the course of talking about these theological problems, we will encounter several feelings which can be dealt with by chaplains from a unique perspective. Shame and guilt are so often mentioned in tandem that many people assume they necessarily go together or are even synonymous. Of course, they do share some characteristics. Both have to do with not being as good as one thinks one ought to be. Both are very common feelings among cancer patients.

The difference is that guilt is the feeling that one has committed some wrong act, either by commission or omission. One has done or even felt something that was not right. What is often labeled as guilt may be the most common feeling we deal with as hospital chaplains. As discussed earlier, most people at least think they have some misdeeds in their past which can come back to haunt them. An unexplainable illness, such as cancer, raises the possibility that the time of that reckoning has come.

However, much of what presents itself as guilt is actually shame. Shame is a more generalized sense that one does not measure up. It is a sense that, on some basic level, one is not good enough as a person. The diagnosis of cancer may make the person aware of this normally dormant feeling. What the patient identifies as guilt may actually be what Burton calls "original shame" (Burton, 1988). This feeling is typified by the patient who was about to be discharged after treatment and said to me, "I don't know if I can go out when I get home. I don't want anyone to see me like this. I'm ashamed of what I have become." Part of this shame is confronting one's own mortality–the feeling that the "flaw" of mortality has been exposed.

Humanist psychology deals with these feelings about imagined or suspected shortcomings by helping people vent them and then by helping people see that there is nothing about who they are or what they have done that justifies these feelings. This strategy works for many people but not for others, especially those who simply refuse to believe that they are good people. The chaplain operating out of the Judeo-Christian tradition does not have to rely on convincing the patient that he or she is good. Through our rituals, prayers, scripture and simply by being there as a representative of God and the religious community, we testify to God's acceptance of the patient as he/she is. Again, we certainly want to allow the patient to vent feelings and to have those feelings validated. However, for us that venting cannot be the end of the process. With the patient who believes in God, our task includes at least an attempt to reinforce the belief in God's unconditional acceptance and irrevocable covenants. To not at least test to see if the patient is open to that kind of reinforcement is to neglect our calling and the unique contribution we have to make in the health care system.

HOPE

Hope is another feeling that has been largely misunderstood in relationship to potentially terminal illness. It has often been perceived as synonymous with denial. Especially in the days when denial was considered to be a state which necessarily interfered with rational decision-making and good coping, hope was considered an irrational impediment to dealing reasonably with serious illness.

In a recent issue of the *Journal of Psychosocial Oncology* (Callan, 1989), David Callan has written a very helpful article on hope as a clinical issue in oncology social work. In comparing hope and denial, he says, "Denial is a defense mechanism that consists of avoiding the facts, whereas hope accepts painful facts but places them in a wider perspective that includes other, more acceptable aspects of those facts. Hope, to be authentic, must be based on reality, taking into account the obvious meaning of a tragic event as well as additional meanings that a person finds more acceptable." Callan goes on to outline three developmental stages for hope. He calls the third stage, "transcendent hope based on meaning." This stage involves meaning which is not dependent on the present situation and which is unaltered by the course of the illness.

Drawing from Victor Frankl (Frankl, 1978), Callan asserts that this meaning enhances the patient's sense of mastery and therefore improves coping.

We as chaplains are sometimes reticent to talk about hope lest we be accused of being one of those pie-in-the-sky religious types who wants to deny a dismal prognosis. We need to remember that true hope embraces reality. We need to understand that as long as it does not cover over reality, hope is helpful in coping. Moreover, as religious people, we have a kind of hope to offer that science does not.

We offer hope that is not necessarily tied to the absence of disease. We offer one system for giving meaning to both life and death which helps to cope with disease but is not dependent on the cure of disease. We in the Judeo-Christian tradition offer a God who wishes people to be well and whole. Again, this is not to say that curing cancer does not matter or is secondary. This is about saying to people that there is meaning to life even in sickness, there is worth to persons even when they cannot "do" anything and there is peace and serenity to be found even in the midst of pain and suffering.

To make this hope real, we must first offer it. We should not play down or gloss over any person's feelings of hopelessness. However, we should actively help them to move beyond that hopelessness into hopefulness. We foster that movement through our words, but also through our presence. One of the great strengths of the chaplain's role is that we can simply "be there." With our presence, we embody and act out the promises of God for God's people. Because people know who we are, they can infer that what we do is motivated by God's concern for them. We represent a God who does not abandon God's people and who never leaves them to cope on their own.

The point of helping people confront the question of how God works in the world is to give them hope. Bringing people to hopefulness should be the thing we do best both by being who we are and by doing what we do. Being a consistent, reliable presence gives people hope that they will not be alone. Putting patients in touch with a God who is loving and comforting gives them hope that they will be able to deal with the pain and suffering that accompanies their disease. We give patients the assurance that they will not experience a spiritual death no matter what happens to their bodies. This faith in spiritual well being enables patients to focus with renewed energy on their physical well being.

SUMMARY

Finally, what are we about in modern chaplaincy? We have successfully shed our old image as a profession that is more tolerated than valued as a part of the team. We have become as skilled in interacting sensitively with patients and family members as any member of the health care team. We have become integrated professionals in the modern hospital.

While maintaining these skills and that place, we need to reappropriate some of the unique features of who we are as people of faith and reintegrate them into our practice. The time when embracing science meant devaluing religious faith has come to an end. We can and must use the strengths of both science and religion to help cancer patients and their families strive for health.

As we continue to grow in using the tools of science to bring people to faith and hope, we need to appropriate some other tools of psychology to help us. As I discussed, the role of assessment needs a great deal more exploration. Research on spiritual issues in coping with cancer is still in its infancy and desperately needs the participation of chaplains. We need the data from this research to help us maximize our patient's ability to use religious faith in their coping.

As chaplains, we will always be on a bridge between science and religion. We will always have to be careful to stay balanced and not to wander too far toward one end of this bridge or the other. To keep our ministry in perspective, we must always remember that science is a method and a set of skills that we use while religious faith is at the center of who we are.

REFERENCES

Berryman, Jerome. "The Chaplain's Strange Language: A Unique Contribution to the Health Care Team," In van Eys, J. & Mahnke, E.J. (eds.) *Life, Faith, Hope & Magic: The Chaplaincy in Pediatric Cancer Care*, Houston: University of Texas Cancer System, 1985, pp. 15-40.

Burton, Laurel. "Original Sin or Original Shame," *Quarterly Review*, 5(4), 1988, pp. 31-41.

Callan, David. "Hope as a Clinical Issue in Oncology Social Work," *Journal of Psychosocial Oncology*, 7(3), 1989, pp. 31-46.

Frankl, Victor. *The Unheard Cry for Meaning*. New York: Simon and Schuster, 1978.

Claypool, John. *Tracks of a Fellow Struggler*. Word, Inc., 1974.

Kushner, Harold. *When Bad Things Happen to Good People*. New York: Avon, 1981.

Sontag, Susan. *Illness as Metaphor*. New York: Farrar, Straus, and Garrow, 1977.

Where Is God for Us?

Jeffery Silberman, DMin

THE SELF AND THE CARE GIVER

The primary responsibility for many professionals in the hospital is caring for others. Most identified with this role is the nurse. Yet, among others, the chaplain, the social worker, and the physician also devote themselves to serving the needs of the sick and dying. Outside of the hospital, counselors, therapists, psychologists, and congregational clergy are on the front line of concern for the homeless, the less fortunate, and those in need.

By and large, the commitment of such individuals who care for others is seen in a very positive light. Our society holds in high regard those who devote themselves to the well-being of others. More recently, however, some have begun to look at the other side of the care giver role. The focus of this recent analysis is the motivation for selecting to do this type of work, as well as the long term effects of these motivations upon the functioning of the care giver.

Clearly, the choices which we make reflect something about who we are and what motivates us. Choosing a care giving career, for example, often reveals the needy side of ourselves. It discloses that we too want to have someone like us available when we are in need.

For some of us, the decision to go into a helping profession is a disclosure regarding our own search for health and wholeness. The struggle experienced in our family of origin may lead to a career in family therapy. A seriously ill sibling may direct one to a medical career.

Another source of motivation for those choosing care givers' professions is the search for love. When as children we strived for the attention and affection of our parents, we felt unwanted or unappreciated. As adults, we were able to offer the care and concern which could earn for us the love and attention we missed as children.

Each of us has a myriad of motivations which led us to our respective careers. Some of us seek to fulfill our neediness; some seek to save others; some of us even seek the power which this work gives us over others. Yet, one important question which faces all of us in care giving professions is whether or not we can care for ourselves even as we do for others.

THE CULTURE OF CARE GIVING

The dynamics of care giving which pose problems for us are not limited to the personal. Our society in general has adopted standards and expectations which can be hazardous to the well-being of the individual care giver. Our institutions from family to schools, churches and synagogues, and hospitals and government, establish unrealistic ambitions for those functioning within them. Our families, for example, are often governed by rules which limit the expression of feelings. Our schools function upon the premise of perfection; the goal is straight A's. Our religious institutions presume the highest moral behavior without regard for individual differences. And then the hospital or congregation or university, wherever we devote the major part of our life's work, asks for more—in effect, devotion and self-sacrifice at the expense of our personal lives. It is truly no wonder that care givers experience burn out. The demands of a lifetime of training from our families, our schools, and our religious institutions compound in the demands of daily life. Many of us burn out; others feel guilty or dissatisfied; still others seek escapes in drugs or alcohol when we feel that we cannot live up to the so-called "normal" way of functioning. When we listen indiscriminately to the cultural message of "work harder, faster, longer, more, more, more," we push ourselves towards sickness and even death.

Why do we opt for such destructive behaviors? What inhibits us from an effective source of help in coping with the struggles of life? One major reason is the expectation which our society seems to create about dealing with problems. Our culture has developed an attitude that virtually demands immediate gratification for all of our needs. As Robert Bellah suggests,[1] we are driven by a belief that "happiness is to be attained through limitless material acquisition." If only we have more of everything, then we will solve all of our problems and be happy. Answers must come at the turn of the dial, the flick of a switch, the swallow of a pill, the ring of the phone, the luck of the lottery in order to provide the solutions to pain, loneliness, deprivation, to any and all suffering.

For the care giver, the problem is usually compounded by the difficulty which he or she has in receiving care from others. The care giver sees vulnerability as something which others may experience. In working so hard to care for others, the care giver forgets that humanity is a quality we all share and that humanity makes us hurt like anyone else. Our humanity gets lost in our striving to meet the privation of others.

THE FAITH OF THE CARE GIVER

At the time when people feel most stressed out or when the burdens of daily routine seem to overwhelm, it is a natural human response to look for help. People who identify themselves as religious typically expect to use the wisdom of their faith traditions to draw comfort and support. Certainly, that is the kind of advice caregivers typically offer those who come to them.

But we know that God is not always the first place toward which we turn in distress. We have many excuses and many alternatives which appear to be more accessible, more real to us in time of trouble. We look to ourselves and ask what can I do? Maybe if I take a day off? We call this a "mental health day." What we are often choosing is an escape from the pressure of work, family, spouse, significant other–from those persons or situations which make our lives stressful, confusing, or problematic at the moment. In other words, we find ourselves confronted with the very concerns to which religion has attempted to respond, and we choose other responses.

To put the problem in other terms, we find ourselves facing the human condition of finitude. If we are basically healthy and sane, we choose a manner of response that is benign and does us no further harm than the stress of the circumstances. If we have lost our perspective or are trained by bad examples, then we can choose other means to cope which may not be so sane or healthy. For example, we abuse alcohol or drugs or gambling or food or sex in an attempt to escape from reality and its pain. It is in the context of our own pain that we struggle to accept and deal with our own mortality.

Our culturally conditioned expectations are in direct contrast to the gradual and patient demands which religion offers us in order to deal with life. In order to be prayerful, to uphold moral principles, to preserve religious values, and to find a place of peace, we must labor diligently. In fact, to venture into institutional religion may yield little that is different from corporate America. The ever-increasing need for financial resources, the strain of schedules and deadlines, the pressure of staffing and interpersonal problems are as common to church and synagogue structures as to healthcare and business enterprises. Yet while institutions of religions function in much the same way as business, the spiritual teachings of religion are neither simple nor easily accessible to the person desirous of gaining comfort from them. These teachings demand time (as, for example, in the Jewish tradition, prayer three times a day), concentrated intellectual effort (as in the learning of the Hebrew language for prayer and study of the sources), and patience (as in the duration of study needed to master the minutiae of Jewish law).

So what should we expect? First of all, we cannot change the expectations that pervade our culture. What we can do is begin with ourselves. And as we do that, we begin to change the world around us, in effect by changing our small corner of it. One well-known application from rabbinic literature is the comment regarding Rabbi Zusya. He stated that when he appears before God upon his death, he will not be asked "Why were you not Moses?" but rather, "Why were you not Rabbi Zusya?" We can only change our world by changing what we ourselves do. In seeking to be true to ourselves, we bring about the opportunity to encounter the Divine within. At the same time, our expectations must conform with reality. Then, we must look to the wisdom of our respective traditions to help guide us on our way.

Typically in daily life, our unrealistic expectations of immediate gratification or financial fantasies inhibit us from experiencing the presence of God in our life and work. God is not magical; nor is God under contract to respond to our every whim; and neither is God an automatic dispenser of good feelings. These simplistic illusions about God leave us with little reasonable hope that God can be present in our time of trouble. Whether in prayer or in our actions, such ideation eliminates the practical possibility of our feeling comforted. Under these circumstances, the only satisfactory result would be a miracle–a highly unlikely, if not impossible option. Thus, we remain blocked by how we view the potential of God's intervention in our lives.

FAITH'S ANSWERS

There are two ways in which religious people may utilize their religious traditions as support and comfort in times of difficulty– two ways in which we can personally connect with God in times of distress. For when we say that we are seeking support from our faith, what we are saying is that we want to be able to feel the comfort and support of God's presence. What we are asking is, "How can God be there for the care giver? For us?" To answer simply, we can encounter God in vertical and horizontal ways. In theological language, God can be experienced in either transcendent or immanent modes.

Among other factors, transcendence ascribes to God the qualities of omnipotence, omniscience, and omnipresence. If we see these qualities only as beyond science and our world, then we miss the possibility that they are descriptive of a God who by virtue of these qualities is available for us.

At this point, we may ask how to establish a relationship with the transcendent God, or, in other words, how do we relate vertically to God? The first option is to use the resources that our respective traditions provide. One obvious response might be "Does this mean that we merely should pray in order to connect with God?" While that is clearly an effective starting point, I am proposing a more fundamental approach: to use the specific techniques which have allowed the great spiritual masters to find an inner link to the transcendent God.

Two prominent tools of the mystics and sages of many religious traditions are meditation and study. To meditate is to focus upon the inner dynamic of self that connects with God. It is compelling because it links with those human features which imitate or come from God. To state this in other terms, we use the method of inner reflection as a bridge to the center of our being wherein resides a "spark of the Divine Light."[2] Commenting on prayer, Rabbi Eugene Kohn provides a useful perspective. He writes, "Many people find prayer difficult because . . . they feel that prayer cannot be addressed to God, that at best it is a form of talking to oneself. But the term 'self' has more than one meaning. It may be used in the sense of 'ego,' the source of egoism and selfishness, or in the sense of 'soul,' the transcendent aspect of the Divine Nature. When we seek communion with God, it is not important whether we address God in the second person as Thou, or think of God in the third person. What is important is that we keep our conception of God before us, and that we endeavor to bring our thoughts and our desires into harmony with our idea of God."[3]

We can also reach "heavenward" in our time of distress by opening ourselves to the wisdom of the past through study. The access to that wisdom is clearly available for all through the inspired texts of tradition. In Judaism, besides the Torah and the rest of Scripture, there is the vast network of rabbinic literature centered around the Talmud, as well as the increasingly accessible Hasidic tradition of stories and legends. These literary sources provide endless gateways into the faith of our ancestors and the wisdom of their beliefs. By learning these disciplines from tradition, we open ourselves to the possibility of God's presence in our lives.

The other mode in which we may find God is the horizontal or immanent realm. The world around us, our religious traditions tell us, is all God's creation. Thus, God's presence should be evident in all that we encounter. The traditional Jew experiences God through the activity of observing *mitzvot* (commandments). Unfortunately, our fashion conscious expectations again often interfere in our identifying God in the world. Particularly in times of agitation, it is difficult to see through the haze of disappointment, suffering, frustration, and pain. But we cannot deny that each of us is blessed with many opportunities to grow and to live, even in the midst of difficulties. After all, we tell that to our patients everyday. Judaism teaches that the discernment of our blessings is enigmatic at times, but not impossible. One story which illustrates this dilemma is told of the Hasidic Rebbe Barukh of Medzibozh:

> One day he was saying grace and repeating the verse, *Vena al tatzrikheni adoshem eloken lo lidey matnat basar vedam*–"May I not be dependent on other people's gifts."
> R. Barukh's daughter Reisele interrupted him. "But, Father," she said, "how can you say such a thing? Do you really wish God to stop people from offering you support?"
> "Only God gives," answered Rebbe Barukh. "But sometimes God uses messengers."[4]

The wisdom of this story is that we cannot always know where and how God is present. Yet the problem remains, how do we apply our good advice to the chaos within our own lives?

First, we have to have a clear idea of what we are talking about. We may ask the question in religious language: What is it that we must have in order to function as children of God? From the Jewish tradition I discern three attributes–a healthy sense of self-regard, humor, and love. Once acquired, these attributes allow us to find God within ourselves and within the world around us. I would like to illustrate each of these from the Jewish tradition.

The first idea–a healthy sense of self-regard–is perhaps the easiest to demonstrate from the Jewish tradition. One of the best known precepts of the great teacher Hillel reads, "If I am not for myself, who is for me? If I am only for myself, what am I? And if not now, when?" The message here is self-evident. It argues: Strike a balance in regard to self and other. The role of the individual is important, but the individual does not subsist alone. It is a wisdom that runs throughout rabbinic thought.

The Talmud relates the following answer to this question: Why did God create only one Adam and not many at a time? "God did this to demonstrate that one person is in himself an entire universe. Also God wished to teach humanity that one who kills a single human being is as guilty as if he had destroyed the entire world. Similarly, one who saves the life of a single human being is as worthy as if she had saved all of humanity'' [My rendering].

The Talmud lists several other motives and concludes with this reasoning: "Lastly God did this in order to establish God's own power and glory. When a maker of coins does his work, he uses only one mold and all the coins emerge alike. But the Lord God created all humanity in the mold of Adam, and even so no person is identical to another. For this reason each person must respect himself. . . ."[5]

The essence of this selection is that we are bound to see ourselves as persons of value. In the context of our work, this often becomes complicated. For we are conditioned to believe that our value is contingent upon what we do and, more specifically, upon what we do for others. This thinking is difficult to change. Yet, it is fundamental to our being able to find God in our lives, especially when faced with problems and pressures. It is this quality that also allows us to see beyond ourselves into the world around us. We might say that a healthy sense of self-regard allows us to appreciate our own divinity. That insight, coupled with a sense of our place in community, brings about the balance about which Hillel spoke, which grounds us and can bring us nearer to God.

The second attribute which offers us pathway to God is humor. Humor is a way of giving us perspective on the problems of life. Jewish humor often puts the miseries of one person into the context of the miseries of the world around him. In that way, life's petty problems don't seem so formidable. Humor tempers the seriousness with which we sometime view ourselves, and we in turn are able to reflect upon life's problems with greater wisdom:

A young man once came to a great rabbi and asked him to make him a rabbi. It was wintertime then. The rabbi stood at the window looking out upon the yard while the rabbinical candidate was droning into his ears a glowing account of his piety and learning.

The young man said, "You see, Rabbi, I always go dressed in spotless white like the Sages of old. I never drink any alcoholic beverages; only water ever passes my lips. Also, I perform austerities. I have sharp-edged nails inside my shoes to mortify me. Even in the coldest weather, I lie naked in the snow to torment my flesh. Also, daily, the shammes gives me forty lashes on my bare back to complete my perpetual penance.''

As the young man spoke, a white horse was led into the yard and to the water trough. It drank, and then it rolled in the snow as horses sometimes do. "Just look!" cried the rabbi. "That animal, too, is dressed in white. It also drinks nothing but water, has nails in its shoes, and rolls naked in the snow. Also, rest assured, it gets its daily ration of forty lashes on the rump from its master. Now, I ask you, is it a saint, or is it a horse?''

Those of us who lose sight of humor lose one of the greatest of God's gifts to humankind. Do we not find God in the smile, the laugh, the cheery story, the feeling of humor? Can God not laugh with us?

The third attribute which brings us in contact with God is love. I am aware that the message of love is over-used and abused by many popular writers. Yet, we are all also aware that our religious traditions have taught the wisdom of love for much longer than most of these "newer prophets." In Judaism, many sources make declarations about love. The *Ve'ahavta* of the *Shema* prayer recited daily states, "And you shall love the Lord your God with all your heart, with all your soul, and with all your might." In this context love is a powerful link with the Divine. This notion is repeated in human terms in the book of *Leviticus* which offers us the Golden Rule: "Love your neighbor as yourself." And when you do, you embrace God and the world. All people, we are taught, are created in the image of God.

The Jewish philosopher Spinoza commented on love in comparable terms when he wrote, "The more love a man possesses, the wider his world becomes until it embraces the whole Creation."[6] The love that a person allows him/herself to experience opens up the world to self and opens up the self to God. In adopting a philosophy of love, we bring together the concerns of humanity into unity and thereby we face them together–together with other people and together with God. It is this that we convey to those we care for when we offer to them a ministry of presence.

Martin Buber related many stories about the Hasidic Sages whose outlook he admired and utilized in his own philosophical work. In the following story, Buber captures an essence of the Hasidic spirit and the meaning of love as a religious attitude:

> A Zaddik asks one of his disciples, "If a Jew arises from his bed in the morning and has to choose in one moment between two ways, the love of God and the love of neighbor, which takes precedence over the other?" The disciple did not know. Then the Rebbe explained: "In the prayer book it is stated, 'Before praying one should say the verse: Love thy fellow as one like thyself!' The true love of God begins with the love of people. And if one should say to you that he has love for God and has no love for people, know that he lies."[7]

In order to find God in our work as care givers, we should realize that our task will not be easy. Yet in the midst of the worst situations, God's presence can be discerned, if we are open to it. In the vertical mode of connection, we may meet God in the soulful search within ourselves. We may apply such traditional techniques as meditation and the study of religious, inspirational, and wisdom literature. In the horizontal mode of connection, the attributes of a healthy sense of self-regard and humor and a philosophy of love provide the vehicles to find God in our daily functioning as care givers. These attributes empower us to expand our perception of who we are, to reflect upon the context of our lives, and to appreciate a unity with the rest of Creation.

NOTES

1. Robert Bellah, *The Broken Covenant*, p. 134-135.

2. Carl Jung has also discerned a notion of the likeness of God in the deepest center of the individual psyche. As Marie-Louise von Franz notes, "According to Jung, . . . the idea of God springs from the reality of the unconscious psyche . . . . It is, namely, everything within us which compels fear, submission, or devotion." (*C.G. Jung: His Myth in Our Time*, p. 153) In other places, Jung suggests that the archetype for God is fixed within each person, and it is only left

for us to find it in the search to discover self. In finding self, we find the God within as well.

3. *Prayer and the Modern Jew* quoted in Louis Jacobs: *Jewish Theology*, p. 193.

4. Elie Wiesel, *Somewhere a Master*, p. 81.

5. *A Treasury of Jewish Folklore*, p. 6 from the Talmud.

6. Quoted in *The Eternal Light*, p. 149.

7. Martin Buber, *Hasidism and Modern Man*, p. 237.

PASTORAL CARE
OF FAMILIES WITH CANCER

Families with Cancer:
Insights from Family Therapy

Laurel Arthur Burton, ThD

INTRODUCTION

"There is no such thing as an individual," iconoclast psychiatrist and family therapist Carl Whitiker is supposed to have claimed. His point, however hyperbolic, was that each person's origins, present and destiny is related in some way to other people. It is a similar sentiment to that expressed long ago by the poet John Donne: "No man [sic] is an island, alone to himself. Each is a part of the main . . ." People are parts of systems and caregivers who work with people benefit from recognizing that fact.

In the past most chaplains have tended to focus on the individual patient. In fact, one of the parents of the profession of modern chaplaincy, once told me that "the great thing about hospital chaplains is that we're different from everyone else on the team; we focus *only* on the individual." Today, however, such an orientation

The author is grateful to Chaplain Deloras Wiems who read earlier versions of this chapter.

seems counterintuitive to chaplains who daily work with people with cancer where the importance of family systems in relation to health and illness behaviors is required information.

The focus of this chapter is on the conceptual framework of family systems and the clinical application of that framework in pastoral practice with oncology patients.

FAMILY AS A CONCEPT IN CANCER TREATMENT

Many meanings may be associated with the word "family." R.D. Laing has said that a family "may be imagined as a web, a flower, a tomb, a prison, a castle" [Laing, 1969]. For many people, families can only be thought of in terms of the relatively recent notion of the nuclear group of persons connected by common genetic material, blood ties and shared history. This view, while it has validity, is not very helpful for non-traditional family groupings such as non-married live-in heterosexual couples (with or without children), same-sex relationships, cooperative living arrangements for elders, etc. Evelyn Sieburg is helpful in furthering an understanding of "family" from a somewhat different perspective:

> Although the family is, in some respects, a unique gathering, it is, in other respects, not unique at all. In addition to its quality of "family-ness," it is also a group, system, a communication network, and a tapestry of interdependent, interpersonal relationships. [Sieburg, 1985]

Given that description, it is easier to understand how each person exists in the context of a "family." When one member of the family is diagnosed with cancer, it becomes evident that all other members of that family are somehow affected.

Chaplains used to think of themselves (much as many physicians did and still do) as standing outside the patient, doing something to her/him, yet remaining personally untouched. A systems perspective reminds us that as careproviders we, ourselves, are a part of the whole system. We do not stand outside it. Not only may we affect patients, but we are affected by them. Further, each of us brings our own history to the pastoral encounter, and in that moment we create some small piece of new history. The story is told of a student chaplain making his first hospital visit. As he approached the room he noticed an unpleasant odor coming from the room. Crossing the threshold he caught the smell full force and immediately felt faint. Remembering some sage advice, the novice careprovider found a chair, and sat, head between legs. As soon as he felt able he nodded in the direction of the patient and made his retreat. Upon his return to the chaplain's office he was told to return to see the patient. With reluctance he again made his way to the patient's room, holding his breath as he entered. This time, before the chaplain could initiate a conversation, the patient spoke: "I'm so glad you came back! You left so quickly I couldn't thank you for the prayer you offered." We never fully know how *we*–with our own history, experiences, preferences and even biology–are affecting the other participants in the pastoral encounter.

It is helpful to imagine a series of concentric circles for each participant who, beginning at the center, has a (1) family of origin, (2) family of current intimates, (3) community family, (4) family of culture, and so on.

Healthcare institutions may also be thought of in similar terms, as Diagram 1 illustrates. Patients with their personal self-systems (1) come from and live in particular family/social systems (2) which together are affected by–and affect–the staff careproviders (3). All of these are now operating in the context of conceptions of health

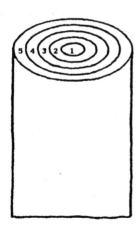

1. Patient/Self System
2. Family/Social System
3. Pt/Fam/Staff System
4. Health/Disease/ Treatment System
5. Policy/Political System

and illness (which may differ from one subsystem to another) within a disease treatment system such as an in-patient or out-patient cancer treatment center (4). Collectively, each of these first four systems are impacted by (5) the policies and politics of the institution and its priorities, state reimbursement policies, and federal programs regarding research initiatives, healthcare funding, etc.

Cancer adds a new element to the above system that must be factored in. For instance, not only does the patient, as a "self," have a personal way of constructing reality related to her/his own genetics, personality, family of origin, etc., but s/he has constructions[1] regarding cancer and its meaning vis-à-vis him/herself. The same is true for the next larger system. Here one observes family stories, structures and styles related to rules, rituals, myths, etc. This system also has a way of constructing and communicating its corporate meaning about cancer. We can follow this through each of the five circles, ending with the larger policy/political system which has its own mode of operation and which has constructed its particular system of meanings–and rules for communicating those meanings) about cancer.

Dr. Bernie Siegel, a Yale surgeon, is noted for his theories about positive imagery and humor as agents for healing cancer. Having worked with a great variety of cancer patients, I have seen several responses to Dr. Siegel's ideas in different subsystems of the larger healthcare system. For instance, I once observed a patient and her family who were excited and hopeful about Dr. Siegel's approach, but who were in a treatment system that believed it to be only slightly better than that of a snake oil salesperson. Needless to say, the differing conceptions about cancer and its treatment were difficult to integrate. On the other hand, I have known chaplains who were so enamored of the gospel of cancer self-help that they sought to apply it to every patient they saw, often spreading the seeds of self-blame among those who did not fully embrace the doctrines being preached (or those whose biological systems did not respond according to the script).

Some patients have told me that "cancer runs in our family and I guess it was just my turn." Such fatalism can be difficult for more aggressively hopeful physicians, nurses and chaplains to fathom. Indeed, it may even run counter to treatments that have an expectation of positive outcome. I worked with one patient for whom cancer was the ultimate threat to personal autonomy and control. Having, because of an early family tragedy, a need to be in complete control, this patient had chosen not to share any information about the disease with family members until it had progressed to its late stages. This was the patient's way of caring for loved ones, by protecting them from painful knowledge. The patient had been classified as "in denial" by some on the oncology team, but a more thorough history revealed the context for a carefully chosen path. The various contexts which are basic to systems thinking provide rich and necessary information for careproviders working with cancer patients.

STRESSORS AND THE FAMILY LIFE-CYCLE

Just as individuals seem to develop over time, so do families. This does not mean that either individuals or families are locked-in to some kind of immutable stage theory. Rather, it means that there seem to be patterns or tasks that are common to people in families at certain times in their lives. For instance Biblical wisdom noted that when a couple unite they must alter the alliances they once had with their parents and form a new alliance with each other. This is one of the movements of the family life cycle. Just how this is done will depend on the culture, ethnicity, socio-economic factors and perhaps gender issues. Middle class WASPS may value separation from their families of origin as the norm for newly coupled people, and thus place a high priority on the couple having their own apartment or house, sometimes at a great distance from the parents. Another culture might draw the boundaries by simply making room for the couple who must now negotiate their own life together in the context of the extended family. In this setting the young couple finds resources, support and companionship. In the midst of these differences, the newly coupled folks are entering a new phase of their life together in which they learn to form a workable duo. At the same time the parents have launched their children into the world and must learn how to relate to them in a different way.

The essential metaphor for the family life-cycle is expansion and contraction or definition and redefinition. Family groups, in general, gain members and lose members. The most familiar example of expansion is the birth of a child when the family is redefined as including three not just two. Over time the child goes to school and eventually begins a life of his/her own. Now the example of expansion has turned to contraction as the family unit begins to shrink or be redefined again, this time in terms of new ways of relating. The place a family is in its life-cycle can be an important factor in how it deals (as a system and as individuals within the system) with a diagnosis of cancer.

During the life of a family, history can play a significant role. Rules for living, stories, myths, etc., are handed down from generation to generation. Beliefs about God and power, freedom and determination, right and wrong are part of these legacies. Also part of the legacy is the biological history of previous generations. "Cancer runs in our family" is not only a belief held by some patients, it may be an astute scientific observation. These historical and genetic elements may be understood as creating *vertical stress* on families. Especially when a family member is diagnosed with cancer, rules, rituals, myths, and patterns that span generations may be triggered. The rule that pain is best dealt with stoically tends to be held in common by a number of WASP families, thus often leaving patients to suffer in silence or risk being further pathologized by the community as "complainers" or "weak sisters."

Horizontal stressors are those that come along over time. They may be developmental–as we have just discussed–or they may be situational, such as an accident, the loss of employment or an untimely death. Imagine what it is like for a family with a mother newly diagnosed with breast cancer and a father who has just been laid off from work (horizontal stressors), who come from several generations of "pull yourself up by your bootstraps" self-reliant yankees who scorn the "undue" expression of emotion (vertical stressors). Patients and families living at the intersection of horizontal and vertical stressors are often in need of a chaplain.

THREE ORIENTATIONS IN FAMILY SYSTEMS

There are many schools of family therapy that could effectively be utilized by pastoral careproviders. However, I believe they can

be classified into three broad categories. These are (1) psychoana-
lytic/psychodynamic, (2) cognitive/informational, and (3) behavioral. By understanding the basic theories of each approach, chaplains
are better able to chose those kinds of interventions that are most
appropriate for a particular patient or family.

Psychoanalytic/psychodynamic orientations to family therapy tend
to focus on historical elements and the role of history in interpersonal interactions. Interpretations and patient insight are important
to this approach. Here unresolved loss issues might be the focus of
work with cancer patients and their families. The psychiatric resident from the Consultation and Liaison service called one after-
noon. "You know something about families, don't you?" she
asked. I said it was an area of specialty and asked what prompted
her question. It seems there was a patient in the Intensive Care Unit
(ICU) who had extensive metastasis and a cranial bleed. She had
been dying for several days. Her children were keeping a round-the-
clock vigil and every time her pressure would begin to drop one of
the daughters would cry out, "Mama, don't go, don't go, we need
you!" and the patient, though apparently comatose, would rally
slightly. The resident asked me to consult with her about the family.
Later, as we stood around the patient's bed I asked the family to
tell me about the woman lying there. They did so in the midst of
fond memories and painful grieving. The story they told involved
the relatively recent death of a beloved maternal grandmother and
an aunt. When I asked who had been the strongest member of the
family in the midst of those losses, they said, almost in unison,
"Mama!" I wondered if there had been other deaths in the family.
The answer brought a litany of near tragic proportions as they told
of the death of the maternal grandfather in a work-related accident
when their mother was young, and the death of the mother's brother
due to a childhood illness only a year later. "But she was strong,"
the family said. "Through all of that, she kept her faith and she
was strong." It seemed to me that such strength was necessary to
survive. It also seemed to me that "strength" could have been a
way of presenting unresolved loss. To my questions about how the
patient had responded to crises the family said she would always
"roll up her sleeves and do what had to be done." "Who's going
to do it when she dies?" I asked. They burst into tears, and one

cried out "But she can't die. We need her too much." There was a predictable flicker on the monitor. "Your mother didn't cry," I asked. "No, never," they said. "How did you learn to cry," I wondered. "Mama always let us cry. She said it was good for the soul. She'd comfort us," they allowed. "And now you are comforting each other," I observed. There was a long silence broken only by sniffles and an intake of breath. "What do you mean," one of the children asked after a time. "Well, it appears to me that your mother is still comforting you by using all her strength to stay alive like this because you seem to need her. I think she's taught you well and that as she dies, you can comfort each other just like she did. I bet she'll be proud knowing that. Why not tell her." Amidst tears and anguished sobs, each of the children touched their mother and told her how they could take care of each other and love each other because she'd been so good to them. I then helped them devise a ritual for saying goodbye and within an hour the patient had died peacefully. Understanding history and unresolved losses can be important in helping patients, families and staff.

Cognitive/informational orientations operate from a stance that assumes families:

> . . . are dynamic evolving systems, always changing and only appearing to be "stuck;"
> . . . are autonomous and therefore cannot be forced to change, and do not need to be pushed around for their own good;
> . . . prefer order and are always seeking to order and re-order their existence;
> . . . will re-order themselves, each in a unique way, in relation to new information.

Brian Lewis writes about this approach:

> [It] "is one of respect and empowerment. There is no judgment made about how the individuals *should* be reacting to the cancer, nor how the family should be functioning. The family is given the message that although they have no control over the fact that a member has been diagnosed with cancer, they do have control over how they react to the cancer–over the

ideas and meanings of the cancer. Somewhat ironically, this attitude of acceptance often facilitates change." [Lewis, 1989]

The following story demonstrates the cognitive/information orientation.[2] I had been visiting a late middle-aged woman of great faith who had ovarian cancer. She seemed to welcome my visits, but appeared to be doggedly fatalistic about her diagnosis. One day she said: "You've got to help me figure it out." "What?" I asked. "For days now I've been trying to think what I have done to make God send me this cancer." I recognized the source of her apparent fatalism. "You are such a faithful woman. How is it that you are so close to a God who would give you cancer?" The question was not resolved that day nor the next, but a seed of suspicion had been planted. As we talked it became clear that the patient's father was both passionate and stern. An authoritarian disciplinarian, he could be both close and warm and harsh and punishing. Her view of God was no longer surprising, either. Over the next few visits I didn't press my agenda, but sought to be supportive. I wanted to create a safe space during a transitional time between the questioning of one image of God and the potential appropriation of another. We talked about many things, but when it came to her big question, I mostly listened. Then one day I asked her how she would evaluate herself as a mother. "That's one thing I'm pretty positive about. I am a really good mother!" I had surmised this myself, having seen her interactions with her offspring. "How did you, as a really good mother, discipline your kids?" I asked. "Well, for one thing, I never hit them or shamed them. We talked things through. I never sent them to their rooms without a meal or any of that stuff. I grounded them sometimes, though. They had to learn that there were consequences to their decisions. Discipline was never a big problem, actually." I questioned further: "What did you do when something unexpected happened, something that wasn't their fault as near as you could tell?" "I just put my arms around them and held them close and we'd cry together . . ." and she stopped. I took her hand as tears began to fall from her eyes. She said, "That's what's happening to me, isn't it? I didn't do anything to make God mad. God's just holding me and crying too . . . like a good mother."

Behavioral orientations, which usually include structural or strategic orientations, focus on the way power is used and, like the psychoanalytic schools, often assume that there is a norm for "healthy" functioning that must be restored. For instance, I was once asked by a hematologist to consult with the mother of a teenage leukemia patient. The mother was refusing the chemotherapy which the physician believed had a good chance of gaining a remission. She wanted, instead, to take her son to a clinic that specialized in macrobiotic diet as a treatment regimen. The rest of the team and I hypothesized that the mother felt terribly out of control. Her reaction of moving in a direction contrary to best medical advice gave her a renewed sense of control. In this treatment system power-sharing was generally encouraged, but the mother seemed to be using her power in a way that could harm her son. Put more bluntly, in our opinion mother was not in a "parent-of-the-patient" role (appropriately interacting with the team around sound medical advice). This related partially to the quick and aggressive way the medical personnel had responded to the leukemia. The hierarchy of the treatment system had been compromised and needed to be restored.[3] We developed a strategy in which I reframed the situation in terms of caring people (both mother and staff) seeking to protect the patient from harm, and in a relatively brief time was able to join with the mother and secure her cooperation in the medically preferred treatment protocol (an appropriate position in the treatment hierarchy), while working with the staff to get mother involved in the ongoing treatment plans (by coaching them to share, carefully and openly, information with her, seeking her opinions and asking her advice). The mother thus experienced herself as appropriately powerful in the care of her child and the physician and team were able to act in a less aggressive way and experience themselves more as partners in the healing enterprise.

Hierarchy, in this model, is generally understood as a positive thing. Some careproviders may have a more negative view of the idea of hierarchy in general, however, thus making it difficult for them to feel comfortable with a behavioral approach. There are, indeed, theologies implicit in each of these approaches, so that those who prefer one over the others may discover a resonance between the approach and her/his own belief system.

I believe that each of these three approaches brings its own benefits, and in fact, has its own problems. I am clearly convinced, however, that the more pastoral careproviders understand each approach and are able to utilize the theory and techniques from whichever school best fits the combination of the patient, the patient/staff/treatment system, and their own style, the more helpful they can be.

HOLDING THEORIES WITH A GENTLE HAND

For many of us who work in healthcare settings, our theories about how things operate are precious to us. They are part of our belief system and we tend to hold on to them tightly. When something doesn't work we may say, "Well, that's the exception that proves the rule," and go on to apply the theory again (rather than alter the theory in some way). As pastoral careproviders adapting the theories of family systems to our work with families with cancer, it can be tempting to choose a single school/theory and apply it to each and every situation. My own experience is that families are not so easily categorized nor treated, and that holding my theory with a gentle hand–and not a little flexibility–empowers greater healing all around.

Two helpful concepts from systems theory contribute to this optimistic stance and help me, as a careprovider, to hold my theories a bit more gently. The first is "circular causality." Social Worker and Family Therapist Lynn Hoffman once used the following analogy to contrast linear and circular causality:

> If you kick a stone, the energy transmitted by the kick will move the stone a certain distance, depending upon the force of the kick and the weight of the stone. But if you kick a dog, the outcome is not predictable on the basis of these forces. What happens will depend upon the relationship between you and the dog. The dog may cower, run away, or bite you, depending upon how the relationship is defined and how the dog interprets the kick. Moreover, the dog's response will also send information back to you. If the dog bites you, you may not kick the dog again. [quoted in Nichols, 1984]

Unlike the traditional linear concept of causality that A causes B (this bacteria caused that infection), circular causality is a way of responding to the age old question "which came first, the chicken or the egg?"

Consider the patient (mentioned above) whose history included a tragedy that, I said, left her with a need to be "in control." That, on the face of it, is a linear attribution. The patient acted in a certain way because of a particular incident in the past. But the situation was far more complex and the explanation far more circular than that. Indeed that early and tragic happening was important. It had led to behaviors which one might associate with maintaining a sense of control. However, there were other factors at play, as well. First, the patient had grown to maturity during the depression, a time that required immense courage, creativity and hard work to endure and survive. Second, as a young adult the patient had built and run a small business that demanded personal attention to its daily operations. Third, the spouse and children had sought (or learned to seek?) stability, strength and guidance from the patient, depending on the patient's advice and consent for most all large decisions. Is any one of these factors the explanation for the patient's response to the diagnosis of cancer? Do each of these flow successively, one from the other, in an orderly way? Can we point to one as causative and the others as adjunctive? I personally don't think so. The point is that each of these factors was a stimulus and a response. Each altered the situation somewhat.

The second systems theory concept that contributes to my optimism about working with families is "equifinality": the same conclusion can be reached even if we start at different places. Imagine taking a trip to Cancun, Mexico. You are sitting on the beach and discover that the people to your right came from Seattle and the people on your left came from New York. You, yourself, came from Michigan. There are three different origins but one destination. Probably everyone flew, but it is likely there were also three different airlines, three different ways to reach the same conclusion. That is one important aspect of equifinality. The return journey illustrates another point about equifinality, namely that when everyone leaves that resort beach, they will start from a common place but reach different conclusions.

Applied to healthcare situations, equifinality helps explain how vastly differing approaches to the treatment of families with cancer can all seem to "work." Whether we start from the treatment perspectives of chemotherapy, surgery, radiotherapy, meditation, or visualization, etc., we can document healing outcomes from each. Likewise, most of us are aware of populations for whom exactly the same treatment protocol is prescribed, but who have widely varying outcomes. Equifinality and circular causality require us always to adapt, rethink and rework our theories and our practices as careproviders and to hold them more gently.

A KEY TECHNIQUE

Whatever the school or theory we as careproviders may espouse, a key technique in the understanding of personal and familial beliefs about cancer and the way they are affecting (and being affected) the family and patient, is "circular questioning." This is different from the usual history taking which tends toward a structured interview format. Circular questions provide information about *how* beliefs and patterns are maintained as well as information about the patient's and family's explanations (*why*) for those beliefs and patterns.

Often a careprovider will hold an idea that suggests that this person or that person in the family is "good" while another is "bad." While it is seldom so stereotypical as that, chaplains and others on the treatment team may reify behaviors or beliefs (such as denial) to such an extent that they focus on breaking through and/or eliminating that behavior/belief sometimes to the exclusion of everything else. Patients and families usually are well aware of the careprovider's position. This means that often chaplains and those to and with whom they provide care are in opposition to one another.

Circular questioning offers a different stance, one of *engaged neutrality*. The careprovider is engaged because s/he makes some kind of emotional connection and is experienced as authentic in the encounter.[4] However s/he is also neutral—as contrasted to pathologizing the patient or family and thus operating in a position of tremendous power imbalance. Brian Lewis says "In many ways the diagnosis of cancer leaves people and families with the ultimate in a sense of lack of control. A therapist who attempts to coerce the family to behave differently, inadvertently usurps even more control from the family and quite literally adds insult to injury" [Lewis, 1989]. This neutrality does not mean operating without a hypothesis, for indeed the purpose of circular questioning is to help the entire system gain information that will either confirm a hypothesis or contribute to altering the hypothesis of some or all members.

When the careprovider asks a circular question it is based on a response to earlier questions. No single person is the focus of the interview. The careprovider moves from member to member[5] thus evoking a constantly shifting perspective on the situation and allowing people to discover the different perspectives others have on the situation.

Some questions the chaplain might ask include:

What's the problem now? It is important for everyone to get the idea that things change over time. Personal and family life cycles alter the demands and expectations on individuals and family members, and at the same time require an acceptance of the shifts in the life cycle. The critical (or terminal) illness of a parent at the stage of family development where children are being launched into the world can lead to an unconscious cancellation of this launching as the teenage children are brought closer into the family circle to deal with the parent's needs during the crisis. While some of this closeness may indeed be helpful, too much over too long a time can lead to a disruption in the family life cycle which may adversely affect all the participants.

Who is most/least affected? While we might assume that only the patient is affected by cancer, in point of fact, everyone is affected in some way, and some more than others. For example, one might assume that a dutiful teenager who has been attentive and helpful during the hospitalization of the mother is affected in only a minor way. Yet when the chaplain asked "who is most/least affected by mom's illness?" a sibling mentioned that this teenager has been cutting classes at school. Eliciting differing perspectives on who is or is not affected provides information to the team and to the family.

How do others react when the patient does X or feels Y? All behaviors exist in a context and as part of a sequence. This question seeks to put behaviors into context and to identify particular sequences. Using this line of questioning, the chaplain discovers that the oldest child is highly reactive to negative news about the mother, and that class cutting is related to increased visiting of the patient and work around the house.

Circular questions such as these not only provide important information to the chaplain, but they offer everyone involved a chance to gain new perspectives on the interface between and among people and the illness.

CONCLUSION

Ministry with individuals will always be a part of the work of chaplains, especially with oncology patients. We can't forget, however, that every individual is a part of a number of larger contexts which s/he affects and is affected by.

Even when the patient seems to be alone, family dynamics may present themselves in the healthcare setting, whether it be during a hospitalization or in an out patient setting. Awareness of the family life-cycle and the nature and role of vertical and horizontal stressors, places individuals and families in a larger developmental context. Choosing from the array of techniques associated with the three general approaches to family therapy provides a flexible guide to interventions. An understanding of systems concepts and theories can, therefore, be an important contribution to the holistic treatment of cancer patients, and it is a role appropriately undertaken by the chaplain.

NOTES

1. The word "construction" here has to do with the idea that people construct their realities through cultural-linguistic symbol systems and thus literally "make meaning" of their experience.

2. I first shared this story in *Models of Ministry* (formerly titled *Pastoral Paradigms*), published by The Alban Institute in 1988.

3. Much of the behavioral [structural-strategic] literature stresses the importance of appropriate power hierarchies. In the medical setting, a sometimes *over*-powering hierarchy, when the power in this vertical structure has gotten misappropriated, the task is to rearrange the structure so that participants are in their given roles.

4. Boszormenyi-Nagy, a more psychodynamicly oriented family therapist, has a phrase "multi-directional partiality" that also catches the flavor and quality of engaged neutrality.

5. This approach may be equally useful in team conferences where some reified belief or pattern of behavior seems to be blocking a more holistic approach to the patient or family.

Cancer and Family Members

Elaine Goodell, PBVM

Kevin's brother, David, had had brain surgery, and it was more than Kevin could cope with. Both boys were athletic, both wanted to be coaches like their father, and so to cope, Kevin continued with his jogging around their little country town of about 1,000 persons. In small midwestern towns–everyone knows everyone, and when they saw Kevin, they would call from the window, run to the door, or run outside and ask, "How's David?" In one of Kevin's rare open moments, he said, "Each day I would jog all over town, and so many people would come out to ask me about David. But no one ever asked me how I was doing." Kevin–and other family members–will forever be impinged and impacted by David's cancer. It is an illusion to consider oneself solely as an individual. As in our story, usually the entire focus is on the patient, and the other family members are assumed to be all right. Personal experience shows that this is rarely true.

David, 18, the oldest of five children, was just entering college but went with his parents to check out his migraine headaches. He was diagnosed with glioblastoma, the most malignant type of brain tumor. Its rapid enlargement destroys normal brain cells and leads to a progressive loss of function. His surgery took place on the day he was to begin college.

When the doctors operated on the cancer on the left side of his head behind his ear, they were unable to remove it all. He and his family were not aware, at first, of how their lives would be changed by the cancer. They were told after the surgery that David had three months to live. That day, his mother, Kay, said, "All hope was wiped out." She continued, "I have heard that one principle of Alcoholics Anonymous is that you have to be all the way down before starting up." She encouraged the family, "We are down at the bottom, so let's start up and let us not plan the funeral."

73

As mentioned, David is the oldest of five children. His siblings are Debbie, Kevin, Steve and Kris who were 17, 16, 15 and 13 years old respectively at the time of his diagnosis. Kay, his mother, worked full-time in the home. Richard, his father, was a high school coach and physical education teacher.

ROLE OF CHAPLAIN

So where does the chaplain enter into all of this?–into the lives of these conflicted patients and family members: Should the chaplain enter? What role does one play? Ernest Becker said, "If I were asked for the single most striking insight into human nature and the human condition, it would be this: that no person is strong enough to support the meaning of his or her life unaided by something and/or someone outside himself or herself" (Becker, 1969). Hopefully, the chaplain is another "SOMEONE" of whom Becker speaks, outside the patient, family, and staff to whom all can turn.

I think of the chaplain in this multidisciplinary setting as a leitmotif. Liszt and Wagner use the leitmotif to hold together some of their compositions. It is a short, recurring theme that through repeated association can identify a person, situation, or thing. It communicates to the listener what is going on with the story. It will appear anywhere in the music and often is unexpected. It's an available tool and easily recognized when used. It is not the main theme of the music and cannot stand alone but makes a valuable contribution in the complex organization of a musical masterpiece.

One of the main purposes of the leitmotif is to highlight the main themes and allow them to be heard more clearly. It bridges the gap between different parts of the piece. Communication issues are probably the most difficult concerns for the family next to the illness itself. Communication is a bridge allowing for interrelatedness. The chaplain's relationship develops from listening and allowing the family member or patient to bring up issues that need to be talked about and heard. Two of our coping mechanisms are talking and listening. Listening is probably the greatest gift we can offer another. The good listener hears, feels, and experiences what the person is sharing, and healing takes place. A good listener connects a person to the world.

The chaplain, like the leitmotif, is first and foremost, a listener. Both patients and family members need someone who can take time, sit down and listen to their stories. They need someone outside themselves, some objective person. Often in the first twenty minutes of a visit the chaplain has been presented with a whole life story—all the poignancy and drama of a real soap opera.

As a channel of communication for patients and family members, the chaplain must realize that each person is probably in a different phase of coping and/or reacts differently; the chaplain must be nonjudgmental and validate feelings of anger, resentment, frustration, and crying, and at the same time assure the person that such are normal responses. David was sometimes resentful and bitter and would refuse to follow directions from the staff. He later said it was important that the chaplain allowed him space and communicated understanding.

COMMUNICATION

Communication is difficult even in the best of times. When cancer strikes, one must decide, "To tell or not to tell?" David's family, in a sense, did not make the choice to share with others, but the choice was made for them when their parish priest appeared unexpectedly at the time of surgery and said, "You are going to play it straight and be open with your family, relatives, and friends." They were, difficult as it was. Normally, this kind of direct intervention might be considered too aggressive and confrontational. However, in this case, the priest presumably had known the family for a while, was familiar with their history, and had a strong relationship with them. Additionally, in the midst of a crisis such as this, a family's decision making capacity may be severely impaired. They may be immobilized and therefore require an outside person to direct them. The leitmotif can add strength to the music around it as well as simply forming a connection.

David's family, up to this time, operated in closed patterns of communication, i.e., information coming in and going out was censored. They were not comfortable with emotions and even frightened of intense emotional display. We are not just speaking of an immediate family of individuals who repressed emotions but of a long standing family history touching generations on both sides.

The family also came from the midwest, a rural state, where crop failures, often year after year, affect entire communities but are stoically accepted by all. Let us also realize that within our own society, open communication is not the norm–deep emotions are generally avoided. These were people who cared profoundly about each other but were overwhelmed by suddenly having to deal with a catastrophic disease. They point up the necessity of assessing and taking into account cultural and familial patterns of coping and communicating.

Both sets of grandparents were contacted by phone and were greatly distressed. They considered it a disease of old people and all would reiterate, "Why not me?" It was especially stressful for the seventy-six-year-old paternal grandfather, for he had never visited a doctor or a dentist in his entire life. When his children were sick, he, himself treated them with home remedies. The maternal grandmother was laid off work the day before the diagnosis, so she immediately went to care for the family; doing was coping for her. The chaplain needs to be aware that the extended family may also be suffering. The chaplain needs to reach out to these people directly or through the community clergy.

Many patients, at the initial diagnosis, tend to become secretively protective and work towards sparing their families and loved ones the devastation they feel. They find it especially difficult to tell children and elderly relatives; they want to protect them. Speaking openly and candidly is usually appreciated by the young and old, for inclusion and mutual exchange is preferred to exclusion and seeming alienation. Personal experience indicates that open communication regarding cancer and its treatment as well as free expression of feelings of anger, sadness, fear, joy, and hope–of both patient and family members–helps to relieve anxieties and contributes towards mutual support and adaptation. This principle also applies if and when dying and death become a reality.

We must also be alert to the family that moves in the other direction and enters into a "conspiracy of silence" where everyone agrees unconsciously or tacitly to keep silent, not to talk about "the elephant in the middle of the room" because they don't want to deal with it or don't know how.

Unfortunately at the time of diagnosis, no one was there to help point out to David's family different strategies of adaptation; the benefits of working as a team for the patient's recovery and their own well-being; the necessity of open communication and looking out for each other in his or her reaction to the stress. In crisis situations, one tends to forget one's own needs, including emotional support and even correct nourishment which is an essential support as well. Although the family was to share the news of David's illness with others and the community, their own habitual patterns of interaction required considerable help and support to change. It took time for David to become open in his sharing with the chaplain. However, he came to the point where he could ask the doctor to call me, thus taking responsibility for his own needs. Richard never came to the point of openly sharing himself, but encouraged others in the family to talk about their concerns with me.

In retrospect, Kay, the mother, tried to talk to family members from the beginning, but was unable to overcome the familial pattern of silence. If she could have been supported in her efforts by someone like a chaplain, she might have been more successful. In this case, the chaplain's role is not simply as a conduit passing information from one person to the next. The chaplain is actively advocating for a certain style of communication and supporting family members who are attempting to be open.

Communication can begin with the physician's relationship to the patient and family. This relationship is so important that it is no wonder the God-image has evolved for the doctor. The family of the individual places a life in the physician's hands. Communication for David's mother also came by steeping herself in all the information she could obtain regarding her son's disease. This can be quite cathartic for the patient and family because it is the unknown we fear. Family can greatly assist the patient and staff. No one knows the patient better than the family and this mutual interaction continues. The family is often more alert to changes in the patient and is aware of possible effects of medication. At one point, David had to go to the emergency room with persistent vomiting. The doctor on duty ordered intravenous hydration. Although Kay insisted that David's arms needed to be wrapped in hot packs before a needle could be inserted into his vein, she was ignored. After repeated attempts by a nurse to insert an IV, Kay screamed for the anesthetist who came and confirmed her story. In another incident over a weekend after David had his shunt inserted, Kay became very concerned about the extent of his vomiting and his lack of gross motor skills. She finally discovered that he was being given a drug to which he was known to be allergic. Again, it took a great deal of complaining and the return of David's regular physician to rectify the situation. Communication with and support of the staff in this regard can be helpful to all.

During David's hospitalization, both he and his mother had questions regarding all aspects of his brain surgery, care, treatment, etc. She encouraged him to do the questioning, but he would not. He said, "That's why I have you here." His mother felt he should assume as much responsibility as possible but in his weakened condition she acted as a go-between even though she preferred he be independent. In some families, a parent will usurp power—even a spouse will continually talk for a patient. Here, a balance was struck, and although she continued to encourage him to communicate, she did not refuse his request.

The chaplain can function as a helpful bridge between the doctor and the family. The chaplain hopefully has a relationship with both parties, understands some of the language and procedures of medicine while being trusted by the family and can listen and talk to both sides.

NORMALIZATION

David's seventeen-year-old sister, Deb, responded to the crisis by wanting to quit girls' basketball and withdraw from being a "Snow Queen" candidate. After realizing his increased stress and torment because of this, they visited and spoke very openly, with Debbie continuing her ordinary activities. David attempted to help her set boundaries since she felt that if he had cancer, she had to suffer. He was saying, "You don't have cancer, I have cancer. I can't play basketball, but you can." No doubt he felt less guilty and she less resentful. It is interesting that in an art therapy session in a weekend family support group, she was the only one of the family to draw sunshine and flowers and to indicate optimism; her two brothers had shadows and closed doors.

In a normal, balanced family, the parents are a responsible, effective, and caring team. The children are dependent on that team for their needs and desires. When one member becomes ill, that role changes, at least to some extent, and the family members see their usual needs and support in jeopardy, especially their emotional needs. Unfortunately, most family members will not think of time management in the crisis, but one parent will assume new responsibilities, along with visiting the ill family member as often as possible and eventually become very tired, stressed out, and almost ill.

In retrospect, David's mother regretfully commented that she allowed her husband and other children to take a second place in her life. She now believes that she had tunnel vision in taking on the whole burden of care for David at the hospital. Although this kind of problem is relatively normal, a chaplain could have helped her gain some perspective on her situation by pointing out the negative consequences for both her and David. Allowing for dual-responsibility at least on weekends could have helped all involved. She also expected in return as much as she was giving, but her husband continued with his coaching and teaching routine as usual; surely he needed to continue financial support of the family. At the same time, however, she needed support from him and viewed his behavior as calloused and uncooperative. In reality, he was coping differently and submerging his suffering in belonging to eighteen organizations.

Four years after David's surgery, when he was in a coma, suffered major strokes, received a shunt, and needed occupational, speech, and physical therapy in order to learn the motor skills all over, his father began to change and realized that work should not be his first priority. Interestingly, in the past few years, the pendulum has swung in the opposite direction and he presently belongs to only one study group. He never did share personal feelings and even while being a vital part of the "I Can Cope" group, his participation was more on an intellectual plane.

His wife admits that a number of times the marriage was in a state of crisis and when they needed to share and work at it, there was simply no time to do so. When a child comes down with a traumatic illness and especially when one parent becomes the primary caregiver, statistics indicate that divorce is a very high probability.

ROLE OF COMMUNITY CLERGY

Church and community also represent a normal relationship for the family and patient. As previously mentioned, the priest representing their spiritual family, immediately connected with them in their crisis and directed them on the road of open communication. Because they followed his advice and went public with their church and local community on the first day, they received tremendous support throughout his illness. The entire community sponsored a "Fund Raiser." Grateful as they were, it was sometimes an embarrassment, especially embarrassing for the siblings who would see the canisters in each store.

This is understandable when we realize that the siblings were seventeen, sixteen, fifteen, and thirteen, and along with David, eighteen, were on the "bumpy" road of adolescence. David was looking forward to independence (and no doubt the parents also) while at the same time wanting security and affection. Also, uppermost for all of them at those ages, was the desire or real need for conformity, to be part of the group—in whatever was said or done. Surely, *never to stand apart* as an object of wonder, criticism—or compassion. David later commented, "When the doctor told me that I had cancer, that didn't worry me much. What bothered me is when he told me they were going to cut off my hair." When his surgery was over, he admitted, "There was a time in the hospital when I held my hunting knife in my hand and thought about killing myself. That was as close as I got."

His concern, as with most teenagers was with his physical image. He sustained feelings of inadequacy, worthlessness, altered self-concept, disapproval, and rejection. He confided, "Some of my friends ignored me. I felt pretty bad, but eventually I just had to put them aside." His siblings, too, had increased social and emotional stresses. They had to continue with school, face friends, and wonder how they really felt about David's cancer and how they would respond to them. In addition, as in many families, the parents focused most of their energies on David and had little left for the siblings. At times I have asked David's mother what Kris, the youngest, was doing at a point in David's illness, and she has no memory regarding her or the activity. Unfortunately, the siblings did not communicate their needs.

As the leitmotif brings into perspective and highlights the other parts of the musical piece that surrounds it, the chaplain can highlight the individuality of each family member. The chaplain can support each family member in fulfilling his or her own needs.

SUPPORT GROUPS

The value of support groups for patients is well documented; however, groups for individual family members and family as a group is also documented positively (Galinsky, 1985; Spiegel, 1989).

The first support group attended by David and his family was exactly that "something mentioned by Becker." It was a turning point for most members of the family and was conducted for a full weekend by the initiators of "I Can Cope." This group was called "We Can, We Can." At first David and his siblings were resistant and whereas the parents had tried all along to respect David's wishes and encourage his independence, they insisted that all attend with the exception of Deb who was in the Snow Queen Contest. After their first hour, David said, "Deb has to attend this weekend at another time and I'll come back with her."

However, each individual is different and Steve, the sixteen-year-old sat in each session with his hat and coat on and with his duffel bag by his side. In one session where each had to relate one positive experience from David's illness, Steve said that if it hadn't been for David's cancer, the family would never have been given free tickets to the Viking game. The remark, however humorous, probably indicated roaring rage rather than gratitude for relaxation.

Neither could the mother find anything positive about the experience at the time; she says now that it was too close to the time of surgery and the resulting trauma. Her positive experience occurred when each family member had to say something positive about the other. David pinned on her, "You're the best treatment for cancer."

The support group served as a catalyst in effecting change in the family. David seemed to pull out of his three-month depression and even though he had passed his three-month prediction of death, he was determined to go back to school, move in with his friends in the dormitory, and drive his car. Everyone was against it and feared for him. He, previous to the Support Group, decided to pull out of the Chemotherapy which at that time was very toxic and debilitating. Both sets of grandparents objected strongly and could not believe the parents would allow such a thing. The parents knew he had to be in charge of his own life and had to "call the shots." They realized that in discontinuing the chemo and having other goals, he instinctively and spiritually knew what was right for him. He listened to his inner being and knew his body best. I might add that the decision about supporting his desire to drive plagued the parents; at first they secretly followed him.

As the leitmotif, the chaplain can support both David and his parents in doing what they both know is right. Although in this case, the doctors agreed with David's decision, in other cases the chaplain may have a role in mediating between medical staff who want to continue treatment and patients who want to stop.

In a family, we cannot expect all to respond to stress in the same manner. Steve, the one with the hat and coat on through all the support group sessions, to this day has never accepted the illness; however, the family members have accepted his non-acceptance.

One of the pointed messages learned in the support group was that family members must be good to themselves. We try to convey that to our families but often it is not heard. Just as David's sibling, Deb, felt guilty about continuing her outside activities and having fun, so it is with many family members of cancer patients or any other illness. It is essential to continue with "fun" activities as previously enjoyed. Exercise and social contacts are all the more important for the well-being of the well. Tensions, frustrations, and resentments are more apt to disappear. It is very important not to feel guilty. Besides talking over coffee or in the cafeteria, what stands out in Kay's mind is when I told her that it was O.K. to laugh. At the time she was horrified and thought it was the worst thing she could do. She says I was the only one who told her such a thing. At another time, she remembers my being with the family in a cramped room in the hospital during a blizzard. What struck her was that I sat down on the floor, was not in a rush to leave, joked with them and simply had a good time.

David's family borrowed money and went as a family on a trip. although David was ill part of the time, it was still a good decision and all participated wholeheartedly.

The leitmotif appears anywhere and availability characterizes the chaplain–even if at the oddest times. The only time David thought he was going to die was the period before his strokes. He wanted me to come and pray for him so the doctor contacted me and I went. The image that remains with his mother is seeing me with David, praying and holding the emesis basin and in our few contacts she still repeats that as a meaningful experience, not only because it represented my total involvement, but because afterwards he immediately went peacefully to sleep and never did vomit again.

I believe it is important to maintain a connectedness (the leitmotif concept), a connectedness back to the issues of illness–and death–where it has occurred. As mentioned, Kay, in each of our visits relates this story and when I last spoke to her, thanked me for allowing her to talk and think about the illness again; most of her family members prefer not to talk about it. When the patient dies, a connectedness with this loved one should continue "down the road" in follow-up visits albeit by telephone. The chaplain as communicator/listener/connector ideally continues in this role after the treatment and death experience and has to be willing to still process the illness with the family. Someone needs to remember the family when others go back to normal activities.

Sibelius, the great Finnish composer, insisted that any great musical composition is religious because it tells a story of life and death. Existential issues will be apparent throughout the entire cancer ordeal for each family and each family member. Grief begins at the time of diagnosis and the "Why's" and "Why Me?" are presented to the chaplain. It is good to talk about their immediate loss or losses and share with them the normal grieving process so they know they aren't the first to endure these feelings and are not having a breakdown.

The leitmotif, functioning as a bridge to connect the various sections of the composition, and the chaplain, also, as a bridge to God, can use prayer, not as a substitute for dialoguing and sharing the family's and the patient's pain, but as a powerful resource when it is applicable. David's mother said that communication, prayer, and hope pulled her through the experience. Prayer, of course, is communication with God. The prayer on her lips each day was from Philippians 4:13, "I can do all things in him who strengthens me."

The leitmotif does not stand alone. I think that it would be impossible to work effectively for patents and families at Memorial Hospital without the trust, support, cooperation, and caring of the Interdisciplinary Team. All patients are admitted to a hospital for diagnosis, treatment, and nursing, but it is in a setting like this that one realizes each person is multidimensional and that true healing includes not only the physical but emotional, psychological and spiritual. This team which is very open with one another confronts the reality of the family situation and plans to do what is best in all aspects of the family's care.

One of the supports offered is hope and this is done from each person's discipline. Hope seems to be programmed into our very beings. When specific wishes aren't realized, families and patients easily adjust and start hoping again.

Some of the hopes of David and his family were realized and some were not. David did not die. He lives alone, frugally on SSI benefits. Since the placement of the shunt and strokes, he is subject to flashing lights in his eyes which precede mini-strokes on the side of his body but then subside. He finished college in eight years but has no job right now. Much of his life is built around denial, e.g., he can't get a job because "they ran out of money," "changed their minds," etc. His social skills are limited and there is an inability to express himself–except when it comes to speaking about cancer. He is an integral part of a cancer support group but needs new goals. He still wishes he could coach and teach and I have suggested to him that he is coaching and teaching. In late 1986, David wrote, "Dear Sr. Elaine, thank you for visiting me and praying for me, and thank you for taking care of Mom and Dad."

Debbie does coach and teach and is close emotionally to David.

Kevin, the runner, is coaching and teaching and never speaks about the illness and seldom sees David.

Steve, who never accepted David's illness still rejects that part of his life. To this day, he cannot stand to be around illness or even a person who coughs. He has done well in his professional life and has received a White House Achievement Award for his work in U.S. Wild Life.

Kris, the youngest, and also close to David, is a physical therapist and volunteers much time to working with the handicapped and the elderly.

Kay, the mother, finished her college degree when David was working on his and had her life on hold for ten years, socially, emotionally, and marriage-wise. Although now she holds down a full-time job, she treasures her time with her husband and makes a special effort to schedule and plan "dates" with Richard. The bonding and relationship is the best of their entire married life.

Richard teaches and coaches in a larger school. His priorities began to change at the time of David's strokes, and in 1986 and 1987 he began to refuse time commitments except to his family. He is active in one Bible Study Group.

I would like to thank the Donovan family for being my leitmotif and for granting permission for revealing their real names.

An appreciation for family dynamics and basic skills in family therapy need to be part of the armamentarium of the modern chaplain. We must be aware as we walk into every room that, no matter how many people are physically present, we are seeing the family as well as the individual.

REFERENCES

Becker, Ernest, *Angel in Armour*, 1969. Paraphrased in Owen-Still, Sally, Spiritual Caregiving, American Journal of Hospice Care, March/April, 1985.

Galinsky, Maeda, Groups for Cancer Patients and their Families: Purposes and Group Conditions. In Sundel, M., Glasser, P., Sarri, R., Vinter, R. (Eds.) *Individual Change Through Small Groups*. Free Press, N.Y., 1985, 2nd edition.

Spiegel, D., Bloom, J., Kraemer, H., Gotthell, E., Effect of Psychosocial Treatment on Survival of Patients with Metastatic Breast Cancer., The Lancet, October 14, 1989.

SPECIAL CONCERNS

Health Promotion in Oncology:
A Cancer Wellness Doctrine

David F. Cella, PhD

A prevalent myth in the cancer subculture is that oncology professionals do not appreciate the human side of cancer. According to this myth, professionals do not care about people, and their lack of caring blinds them to the richness and power of the human body to heal itself. Logically, then, oncology professionals would not support wellness programs that try to mobilize the human spirit and empower it to take self-improving action. Patients would threaten the health-care empire by asserting that they have personal responsibility for their health, that they control their destiny by living a healthful lifestyle, and that they reject the passive-patient role in favor of an active-participant role.

In my contacts with more than 100 oncology practitioners, I have not uncovered any significant substantiation of this myth. Only a handful of cancer professionals object to our efforts to empower patients and their families by teaching relaxation, imagery, and communication skill. Our goal is to help patients participate more actively in their treatment and to reject passivity when it does not

This article was previously published in *Journal of Psychosocial Oncology*, Vol. 8, No.1, © 1990 by The Haworth Press, Inc.

serve them. At first glance, a passive, compliant patient may appear to be easier to treat then an active, involved one. But that illusion is often shattered by a passive patient who suddenly becomes crucial to effective clinical management. Because cancer is among the growing ranks of chronic diseases that cannot be managed without the patient's participation, oncology professionals typically welcome active, informed patients.

A MODIFIED APPROACH TO PROMOTING WELLNESS

In our efforts to promote wellness in cancer survivors, we are usually unwilling to offer information beyond available research data on the topic—especially when responding to direct questions from patients and family members about the benefits of a positive attitude or the importance of imagery in the healing process. Nobody knows the answers to these questions. We suggest no cures or panaceas; instead, we teach skills that return control and dignity to the person with cancer. Our promotion of wellness is modified with a mild dose of realism to offset some of the hazards of overstated claims.

Our refusal to reach beyond available data may explain why our approach to promoting wellness is popular with health professionals. We promise no benefits, and we do not seek to inspire with anecdotes about other people. (Most patients have already heard these anecdotes anyway.) We do, however, seek to inspire people with a sense of their own personal opportunity to develop. We assess their level of need and create an atmosphere in which the necessary skills can be taught and health promotion is encouraged. The skills we teach include relaxation training, guided imagery, assertiveness training, and problem-solving ability. Because the application of these skills depends on the patient's needs and wants, our approach is closely tied to the empiricism of clinical psychology and related disciplines.

"IS MODERATION EFFECTIVE?"

Because our approach runs a low risk of promoting false hopes or unrealistic convictions about cure, the opposing risk may be more relevant: Does a "modified" approach to promoting wellness fall short of what people seek because it dilutes the message? Unfortunately, only beliefs, without supporting data, are available to answer that question. At times, our approach may seem inadequate to meet the needs of wellness seekers. Perhaps it is analogous to chemotherapy, the concentration or intensity of which has been reduced and thus is less effective than more aggressive treatment.

In my opinion, the pros and cons of training in stress management cannot be debated with cancer patients without acknowledging the extraordinary popularity of mind-body approaches to cancer treatment (Anderson, 1988; Siegel, 1986; Simonton, Matthews-Simonton, & Creighton, 1978). The extent of their popularity is intimidating, perhaps ominous, given the dearth of supportive documentation behind them. The references to anecdotes and unpublished research that abound in books, speeches, and audiotapes create the impression that we know far more than we actually do and, at times, even suggest that a threatened establishment is squelching "the truth."

Thus, two distinct phenomena are interacting today. The first phenomenon, to which we link ourselves, is a set of preliminary, suggestive studies that encourage the trained clinician to teach established health-promotion skills to motivated people who have cancer. The second is a more cultural or even religious one in which local and national "evangelists" preach inspirational messages to interested followers. What is being preached is a message of love and hope that capitalizes on exceptions to the rule as evidence that everyone can expect a miracle. The lectures, books, and tapes of these evangelists are invigorating and enriching and provide a sense of vitality and optimism, but they rarely teach new information or skills. Some of the evangelists' suggestions are misleading or deceptive; others are more benign.

The spate of books and tapes and the sell-out crowds at local lectures attests to the greater popularity of evangelists than of clinicians who teach stress-management skills. But we who practice this more mundane and detailed stress-management approach must reckon with the other phenomenon because patients often come to our offices seeking more after being inspired by a book or lecture. Interestingly, few of these patients are willing to commit the time and money required for a stress-reduction program.

The untempered promotion of any system of beliefs incurs a serious risk. Doctrines can easily turn into dogmas that are arrogantly or authoritatively asserted without proof. Any good principles can be undermined by a vanguard of opportunistic zealots. Indeed, we have all witnessed the exaggerated and inflated claims of practitioners of holistic health programs and alternative therapies, and we recognize that these programs risk alienating the health care establishment and patients alike by overstating their benefits. As a result, we risk losing what is good and useful from the holistic health movement.

At issue here is the question of whether "holistic" oncology can be practiced in moderation or whether moderation of the message somehow removes its healing power. If hope "heals" by fostering faith in cure–in other words, if faith-healing is a teachable commodity–must that faith be unbridled? Must a person hope for and believe in total cure, or can that person hope with equal vigor for some approximation? What is the difference between "heal" and "cure"? If heal means to make whole or complete and cure means to eliminate disease, then heal is a broader term that, to many, implies cure as a component part. To *expect* cure of metastatic disease as the end product of any therapeutic effort, whether that effort is biological or psychological, is excessively ambitious. To *hope* for cure is natural and human. If cure is not attained, as it usually is not, then physical decline and death do not signify failure. The expectation of cure (called "false hope" by some) is not necessarily fostered by promoting hope.

The Importance of Direction

This is the challenge to the health promoter; to encourage optimism, hope, laughter, and whatever else might improve a seriously ill person's quality of life without burdening that person with guilt or, worse yet, with a hollow drivenness toward the unlikely. At times, some redirection, including a return to the essential tenets of stress reduction, is clearly necessary.

I am reminded of a middle-aged executive I once met. He had metastatic lung cancer and was determined to be an "exceptional cancer patient" (Siegel, 1986). His resolve to succeed at this goal was exactly like his earlier resolve to succeed in business, a success he obtained through determination, hard work, and lust for the pleasure of success. With his classic Type A personality–driven, hurried, overextended, and thriving on it–his approach to guided imagery was predictable. He devoted himself to guided imagery fully, embracing its possibilities. His goal was crystal clear: to shrink his tumor completely by combining imagery with traditional treatment. He religiously scheduled three visualization sessions per day. Because his daily work schedule was so tight, he decided to drop the relaxation component so he could more quickly get to the visualization, which he perceived as the central healing agent. In short, he deprived himself of the stress-reducing benefits of relaxation because he felt too much pressure to get to the visualization. His drive to participate in the healing process became hollow because he lost touch with the main purpose of the exercises–to lower stress and regain a feeling of control.

The Medical Mainstream

Hoping for miracles is a familiar concept to oncology professionals. In untold ways, both directly and indirectly, patients communicate to their physicians and nurses that they "don't want to hear bad news." Few oncology professionals can honestly say they have never knowingly misled a patient, either by omission or commission. This deception, arising from a benevolent effort to protect or preserve hope, usually encourages patients to inflate their prognosis.

In this article, the discussion takes the following position: No essential healing component is lost when efforts are made to mobilize cancer patients toward healing themselves in a way that respects *all* that is unknown about health and illness. Many alternative cancer "cures" are marketed by capitalizing on the fact that traditional medicine does not have "the answer." Ironically, these alternative approaches may themselves be presented as that magic bullet. The bottom line is that nobody has a cure for most forms of cancer. The heroes among us are those who promote as much dignity and wellness as possible. Telling people for whom no further treatment is available that they might as well go home to die deprives them of dignity. Suggesting an alternative treatment as a cure that has been neglected or suppressed by traditional medicine is insensitive and unethical because vulnerable people are all too ready to accept this as gospel. Such a suggestion essentially fosters a faith in the underworld borne of desperation.

CANCER WELLNESS DOCTRINE

Our doctrine for cancer wellness is a set of principles or beliefs that can be taught to and then embraced by people with cancer. The word doctrine derives from the same Latin word (*docere*, meaning "to teach") as the word doctor. Indeed, the ideal patient looks to the doctor as being more of a teacher than a healer because healing is a process that is larger than doctors themselves. Healing refers to restoring wholeness or unity in the body, a process that can only be managed and interpreted by the patient. A good doctor teaches, recommends, and cares for the patient. A good patient strives for healing or a return to feeling whole and healthy. This striving is usually facilitated by listening to and following the doctor's recommendations. If a patient feels that these recommendations and the general treatment plan are not maximizing his or her chances for healing, the effectiveness of communication within the doctor-patient relationship needs to be reviewed.

The cancer wellness doctrine currently consists of eight central beliefs, each of which is modified and, at times, tempered in ways that attempt to clarify its limitations without stripping it of its power. Embracing these tenets along with their qualifiers may be even more empowering than blanket acceptance of unproved beliefs because it facilitates better collaboration with the treatment staff.

1. *Belief: My health is my responsibility. Modifier: I did not cause my disease.* People who take responsibility for their health and general well-being are better at combatting illness than those who do not. Believing that one can take responsibility for one's health implies a feeling of personal control. The term "health locus of control" refers to where people lie on a spectrum ranging from the belief that their health is largely within their control (internal control) to the belief that their health is determined by luck (chance) or by health professionals (powerful others). Studies show

that a strong belief in personal control over a health-related situation is associated with improved psychosocial as well as medical outcome (Wallston & Wallston, 1978; Wallston, Wallston, & De-Vellis, 1978). Anything that promotes a person's belief in an internal locus of control will help that person take responsibility for the changes needed to get well.

. The risk of promoting a belief in an internal locus of control is that some people will think or, as we have often observed, be told by a well-meaning friend or relative that they caused their disease. Their attribution about cause takes the following form: "Since I am responsible for my health, and I know I recently subjected myself to stress, did I bring on my disease? Am I to blame for this cancer?" The answer to these questions is a resounding no! Because we know very little about how and why people get cancer, to suggest that people bring it on themselves is unconscionable.

Books such as *Love, Medicine and Miracles* (Siegel, 1986) may inspire people, but they leave confusion and misapplication in their wake. The fact that spontaneous remission occasionally occurs, even when the disease is so advanced that most would consider it to be terminal, is an interesting and provocative reality. Dr. Siegel and others appropriately suggest that we do not spend enough time studying these successes. If we did, we might learn more about the origins of seemingly miraculous remissions. However, our current lack of answers lures many of us into believing that cancer survivors are people who fight for their recovery. This interpretation fulfills a common human need to feel that we can control situations which are actually beyond our control and that the world is basically fair–a place where good things happen to good people and bad things happen to bad people. However, many of us have seen too many fighters die and too many passive patients do much better than anticipated to believe this oversimplified explanation. Indeed, small subgroups of patients and professionals have countered this oversimplification with the following battle cry: "Stop blaming the victim" (Blech, 1989; Ferrar, 1989).

2. *Belief: I will always have hope. Modifier: What I hope for may change over time.* Hope is a valuable commodity. Without it, a certain amount of depression is inevitable. In fact, because so many indicators of depression are contaminated by the effects of

disease and treatment, hopelessness is a valuable clinical indicator of depression in the medically ill (Cella & Perry, 1988). Fortunately, most people are resilient enough to find something to be hopeful about. Our role is to help patients find the appropriate level and kind of hope. For example, if a patient comes to us with unrealistic expectations, such as hope for complete remission of metastatic disease, we do not try to dispel his or her belief in this possibility, nor do we overtly reward that belief by elaborating on unproved ways to bring about remission. If a patient is in despair, we do not encourage that despair, nor do we respond with only a sad, empathetic nod. We struggle with the patient to understand the despair and its function; then we attempt to help the patient discover alternatives to that despair. If hope for cure or remission is no longer tenable, improved palliation, physician-patient communication, family relationships, and personal satisfaction may be the goals.

3. *Belief: My doctor and I are partners. Modifier: We both have things to learn.* People who enter the treatment arena with some sense that they have valuable, meaningful information to give their physicians are generally easier to care for and usually receive better care. The patient's challenge is to learn enough about the physician's personality to see the best way to deliver that information. Such information clearly helps the physician work more effectively, and much of that information–particularly about symptoms and side effects such as pain, nausea, and fatigue–cannot be validly measured without the patient's input.

The past few decades have seen attempts to reverse centuries of socialization in which patients were encouraged to accept medical care passively and "patient-ly." Some patients present their bodies for treatment as if they are specimens with an unwanted disease. Such patients apparently assume that the physician can divine a diagnosis and develop a treatment plan without their help. Parsons (1965) used the term "sick role" to describe patients who relinquish personal responsibility for managing their medical care. Dependency, helplessness, and depression are consequences of adopting this role.

4. *Belief: Death is not failure. Modifier: Personal dignity and quality of life are better measures of success.* We all die. If success is measured by living forever, we are all doomed to fail. Although

it sounds callously self-evident to say this to a person who has cancer–especially to one who is afraid of dying–the statement is true and, if discussed in its complexity, can replace panic with perspective. Also, most people are not dying in the moment. They may have an incurable disease, but it can help them to change their perspective–to see that at this moment, they are alive and doing well. Their goal can be one as simple as maintaining their well-being.

For example, a 61-year old man with prostate cancer–a professional with a doctoral degree who was educated in the rigors of the scientific method–inquired skeptically about the value of relaxation and visualization techniques. This patient was a self-proclaimed realist, perhaps a euphemistic term for a pessimist who views the half-filled glass as half empty. He felt anxious about the prospect of dying from his disease and wanted to know what had been scientifically demonstrated to benefit patients who had this disease. He was secondarily terrified of impending pain, which he assumed to be inevitable because an oncologist once asked: "So, do you have any pain *yet?*" He was desperate enough to seek advice from a psychologist about stress-management techniques but leery of being given "false hope." Such patients are unlikely to embrace false hope; the risk is that they will not allow their armor of belief to be penetrated by nonscientific possibilities.

Work with "realists" typically focuses on cognitive therapy to alter beliefs that obstruct avenues toward improved well-being. Efforts to remove obstructions to hope frequently involve confronting the idea that death is failure. The objective is to replace this idea with one that holds personal dignity and quality of life as more indicators of success in life. Unlike death, which is inevitable, personal dignity and quality of life can be manipulated and controlled.

5. *Belief: Cancer provides me with an opportunity. Modifier: I don't have to be grateful for that opportunity; I didn't need it.* For most people, cancer represents a crisis. Confronted with the prospect of mortality, priorities shift, and confusion about basic aspects of identity or lifestyle may develop. The crisis may lead to significant rethinking about the value of one's career; the importance of family; or more personal, perhaps spiritual, issues. Although most of us are trained to think of a crisis as a negative phenomenon, its

purest definition, as derived from its Greek ancestor, means "turning point." The opportunity for change emerges in any crisis, and because few people live their lives exactly as they want to, cancer can motivate people to confront and change preexisting undercurrents or undesirable aspects of themselves or their lives. Although many people fear change because it requires both effort and confrontation with the unknown, efforts to change can be energizing in the long run.

Any significant stressful event, positive or negative, can stimulate change. For example, a healthy young woman might decide to abandon her career and travel around the world for a year, working at menial jobs to support herself. Her experience, which she perceives as extremely positive, is also likely to be highly stressful. Essentially, she has placed herself in a personal crisis; during this year of change, she is likely to reach at least one meaningful turning point in her life.

Many other stressful events would be more welcome than cancer as stimuli for change; for example, losing a job, getting married, or having children. Thus, we arrive at the modified statement: "Cancer provides me with an opportunity. I don't have to be grateful for it; I didn't need it." No patient deserves to be asked, "Why do you need cancer?" Nobody needs it. A better question is: "Now that you're stuck with cancer, how can you make the best of it?" Opportunities for humor emerge with this line of questioning, and, although laughter may not be the best medicine for cancer, it never hurts.

Encouraging people to make the most of their situation is extremely important. Many of them are ready to be shown how the challenge of cancer can teach them about themselves, their family, and their friends. People can learn to become opportunists, capitalizing in some way on their illness. A young man with metastatic colon cancer once bragged that he planned to "use" his cancer diagnosis as a handicap that would enable him to advance in his business. His resolve turned a bad situation into an opportunity.

6. *Belief: I am willing to change the way I deal with stress. Modifier: The past is unimportant unless I make it so.* A clear link exists between stress and the immune system (Ader, 1981; Borysenko, 1987; Levy, 1985). A clear link also exists between impaired

immune function and the development or progression of cancer (Culliton, 1989). However, the leap from the first statement to the second, which suggests a connection between stress and the initiation or progression of cancer, remains primarily one of faith (Fox, 1983; Levy, 1985). Nevertheless, the idea that previous stress can contribute to the development or promotion of a patient's tumor is widely touted. We never ask people to reflect on past stressful events that might have led to the onset or progression of their disease because doing so would imply the existence of strong evidence for causality. Because this causality has never been proved, initiating such a discussion seems unethical.

If a person's reflections on past stresses (e.g., a bad marriage, personal losses, a dissatisfying career) mobilize that person to take positive stress-reducing action, those reflections are advantageous. Nobody would question the benefit of adopting a healthier, less stressful lifestyle. However, reflections that focus on personal remorse or blaming of others serve little purpose and are best discouraged. A person's self-defeating focus on the past can be confronted by asking what purpose it serves. If a person's espoused purpose is to prevent future stress, then he or she can be mobilized to redirect the focus from the past to the present and future. If a patient or family member cannot let go of the past and theories about its influence on the cancer diagnosis or progression of the disease, then that past will obstruct rather than facilitate progress in managing stress.

7. Belief: Cancer is a family illness. Modifier: Therefore, my family needs my attention now. Although cancer as a disease affects one's body, cancer as an illness pervades the entire family network. Sexual functioning (Andersen, 1985; Schain, 1988), intimacy (Gates, 1988), and parent-child relationships (Lichtman et al., 1984) are affected by cancer. Unless these cornerstones of social functioning receive attention, relationships may drift irreparably apart. If this drift occurs at crucial moments, it may have a detrimental effect on clinical care and decision making.

Consider an extreme case in which a patient is deteriorating physically and mentally: Because nobody wanted to challenge the patient's sense of hope, perceived (perhaps erroneously) as fragile, the subject of resuscitation was never discussed. In a collusion of benevolent paternalism, the family and the physician have agreed, often implicitly, not to mention that possibility. Now, the need to decide has arrived: The patient is confused, perhaps even comatose, and the physician asks the family for a decision. The family must now bear the burden of this decision, perhaps not knowing what the patient would have wanted, because everyone avoided the subject earlier. This extreme example, which occurs fairly regularly, points out the need to include the family in the cancer patient's care. Including close family members in clinical decisions is important, if for no other reason than to avoid later misunderstandings and gratuitous burdens.

8. *Belief: I have the power to make a difference in my care. Modifier: I need to look within myself for the proper direction.* There is no single approach to wellness. Even if the treatment plan includes only relaxation training, at least nine different approaches to this training have been proposed (Smith, 1985). Finding the ideal approach for each individual takes time. The important belief to promote is that people have the inner ability to make a meaningful difference, that the direction of change must come from within the person who has made a commitment to change.

Some patients who enter our offices want to learn how to visualize cancer cells and a healthy immune system that attacks them and flushes away the waste. We do not promote this practice unsolicited because we believe that promoting unproved remedies is unethical. However, when a patient brings this request to us after reading or hearing about it, we incorporate it into our general stress-reduction plan because the patient presented it as a goal. Over time, it becomes obvious which patients are genuinely interested in continuing this imagery theme and which ones would prefer to move on to other areas they perceive to be more fruitful. The task of the therapist in promoting wellness is to make this discovery safe and possible.

CLINICAL SUBTYPES

The cancer wellness doctrine and the general approach to promoting to wellness were derived from, and thus can help identify, at least four different subtypes of cancer patients who will request wellness promotion: realists, opportunists, zealots, and fighters.

As was discussed earlier, realists assume that the odds are against them. Their loved ones describe them as pessimists and often push them to see a consultant about wellness. The therapeutic goal with realists is to clear the obstructed path so they can begin to feel genuine optimism or hope. The risk of promoting false hope is dwarfed by the risk of alienating the realist into devaluing the treatment.

Opportunists want to reduce daily stress but are generally unwilling to commit the energy that makes it happen. If commitment comes easily, with a discussion or two, the effort may be worthwhile. If not, little has been lost. Either way, the health promoter rarely sees the opportunist again after the first session or two. The cigarette smoker who refuses or is unable to quit and then presents for wellness promotion after blaming the cancer on stress is an opportunist. The request for stress reduction or imagery training helps maintain the smoking habit, which obviously is more dangerous to the patient than stress.

Zealots, who are relatively rare, believe passionately in the power of the mind to heal the body. Their conviction is often so strong that it makes professionals feel uncomfortable. However, their zealotry often masks an underlying anxiety. The flurry of activity and the intensity of the drive toward healing and imagery are usually defenses against dealing with the issues of suffering, death, and dying. Rather than discuss their fears in an effort to gain control over them, anxious zealots force an awkward control over those fears by transforming them into mental images that presume to heal.

For example, a woman with metastatic renal cancer who requested a consultation with me said she intended to beat all the odds and live a long and full life. At first, she was hauntingly convincing in her insistence. Within days, however, her almost arrogant insistence changed to pathetic groping for direction as she lay in her hospital bed, insisting on cure. She died quickly, perhaps mercifully, for she apparently never confronted the fears she seemed so desperate to avoid.

Fighters, by far the most common group of patients seeking wellness promotion, are adaptive copers who are genuinely mobilized in a productive, self-improving direction. Like zealots, fighters believe in the power of the mind over the body, but they seem to have the ability to distill useful messages from among those that appear in the popular press and discard messages that are either nonsensical or unhelpful. Fighters may need skill training, but they generally do well without significant cognitive restructuring because they have already learned the art of attending selectively to useful beliefs.

CONCLUSION

Health promotion in oncology has become popular, largely because recent advances in psychoneuroimmunology have rekindled the belief that people with cancer can exert personal control over their destiny. This belief, perhaps premature from a scientific standpoint, is long overdue in the eyes of the average recipient of health care. As mental health professionals who work with people with cancer and their families, we are obliged to attend to and promote this drive for personal control and wellness. We are equally obligated, however, to maintain an objective perspective regarding the current status of the mind-body debate in oncology. This article has presented a doctrine for promoting wellness in oncology that represents an attempt to walk the line between ambiguity in the current state of knowledge and the clinical demand for health promotion services.

REFERENCES

Ader, R. (Ed.) (1981). *Psychoneuroimmunology.* Orlando, FL: Academic Press.
Andersen, B.L. (1985). Sexual functioning morbidity among cancer survivors: Current status and future research directions. *Cancer,* 55, 1835-1842.
Anderson, G. (1988). *The cancer conqueror.* Waco, TX: Word, Inc.
Blech, B. (1989, January/February). Don't blame the victim. In *Surviving!* (a newsletter for patients, pp. 10-11). Stanford, CA: Stanford University Department of Radiation Oncology.
Borysenko, J. (1987). *Minding the body, mending the mind.* Toronto, Ontario: Bantam Books.
Cella, D.F., & Perry, S.W. (1988). Depression and physical illness. In J.J. Mann

(Ed.), *Phenomenology of depressive illness* (pp. 230-237). New York: Human Sciences Press.

Culliton, B.J. (1989). Fighting cancer with designer cells. *Science,* 244, 1430-1433.

Ferrar, C. (1989). Stop blaming the victim. *Cope: Oncology News for Professionals,* 3(4) 46.

Fox, B.H. (1983). Current theory of psychogenic effects on cancer incidence and prognosis. *Journal of Psychosocial Oncology,* 1(1), 17-32.

Gates, C.C. (1988). The "most-significant-other" in the care of the breast cancer patient. *CA–A Cancer Journal for Clinicians.* 38(3), 146-153.

Levy, S. (1985). *Behavior and cancer.* San Francisco: Jossey-Bass.

Lichtmann, R.R., Taylor, S.E., Wood, J.V., Bluming, A.Z., Dosik, G.M., & Liebowitz, R.L. (1984). Relations with children after breast cancer: The mother-daughter relationship at risk. *Journal of Psychosocial Oncology,* 2(3/4), 1-19.

Parsons, T. (1965). *Social structure and personality.* Glencoe, IL: Free Press.

Schain, W.S. (1988). The sexual and intimate consequences of breast cancer treatment. *CA–A Cancer Journal for Clinicians,* 38(3), 154-161.

Siegel, B.S. (1986). *Love, medicine and miracles.* New York: Harper & Row.

Simonton, O.C., Matthews-Simonton, S., & Creighton, J. (1978). *Getting well again.* Los Angeles: J.P. Tarcher.

Smith, J.C. (1985). *Relaxation dynamics: A cognitive-behavioral approach to relaxation.* Champaign, IL: Research Press.

Wallston, B.S., & Wallston, K.A. (1978). Locus of control and health: A review of the literature. *Health Education Monographs,* 6, 107-117.

Wallston, K.A., Wallston, B.S., & DeVellis, R. (1978). Development of the Multi-dimensional Health Locus of Control (MHLC) Scales. *Health Education Monographs,* 6, 160-170.

Caring at the End of Life

Mary T. O'Neill, RSHM

PART 1

The following remarks are addressed to persons who are on the "caring" side of this equation, rather than on the "end of life" side. However, I hope to emphasize the connection and relationship that we're about as we work towards understanding, journeying with and being companion to those persons who are at a major junction/crossroads in their lives. In this way, I hope we can all gain new insight and understanding into ways we can be available and respond to their needs.

Being in a position of caring for someone at the end of life calls for someone who can be a healing companion. A "healing companion" helps a person move towards inner freedom, integration, wholeness. It entails bringing all of who they are into harmony with what is happening in their lives at this particular time. Obviously, this touches all aspects of the person.

"Healing" is not the same as "curing." To "cure" is to change the situation, to rid the person of the symptoms of the disease. To heal, on the other hand, is to help the person move through what is causing distress, dis-ease in the person's soul (the entire realm of the person's thinking, feeling and behaving). This involves working with the person's thoughts about self, the hopes, dreams, aspirations, and fantasies. It involves being with the person in his/her fear, anger, anxiety, guilt, etc. It means standing with them in their concerns about good/bad ways of living and behaving and relating.

Facing death throws a person into crisis–and instead of being life-giving, this crisis creates dis-ease and emotional pain and can easily disorient the person in relationship to self and the world. It calls them to reevaluate themselves in all aspects of their being.

Healing in this instance means being with the person in such a way that he/she can move through the crisis, work through the situation and struggle and come to a place of deeper wholeness and ATONE-MENT with self.

The caring "companion" truly stands with a person in such a way that he/she can touch the deepest core of self. The companion sits with and tastes the broken bread of struggle and distress that cause the dis-ease. This makes for the kind of companionship that can be deeply healing even when there's no hope for a cure of an illness or reestablishment of a loss through death or separation of any kind.

Who is the person who enfleshes what healing companionship is all about? The most essential characteristics is that this be someone who has worked on his/her own integration of body, mind and spirit. A person who knows and understands the road maps from the inside can have profound respect for and understanding of another in crisis. It is someone who is a Wounded Healer, to use Nouwen's words. Nouwen says: It is the "wounded healer" who is willing to put his/her own faith in doubt, his/her own hope and despair, his/her own light and darkness at the disposal of others who want to find a way through their confusion and touch the solid core of life" (p. 39, Wounded Healer). It is hard to remain near pain, most of all when the pain is an anguish for which we feel we can do nothing. We are wounded healers, caring for wounded persons.

The task, then, of the healing companion in assisting another in search for meaning and direction is to be real, i.e., to know yourself, and to reflect deeply on the personal issues and vulnerabilities that get touched, to understand your own dynamics and how these are operative in ministry. This person also must be professional, i.e., have an informed and well-developed sense of personal, pastoral and professional identity.

Dying cannot be avoided or shoved under the table, nor should it be taken for granted that everyone knows how to face the end of their lives. In fact, not many people know what to do when faced with the threat of death. I would consider it quite normal to feel isolation, confusion, fear and great turmoil. With no one to care to guide them through this crisis, they risk staying lost in their confusion and, consequently, suffer more than necessary. Many in our society would agree with Woody Allen when he says, "I'm not afraid to die; I just don't want to be around when it happens." Those who face death desperately need the companionship of someone who is not afraid of them and their situation. They need someone willing to hang in with ugly feelings, someone willing to listen to questions which touch the core of this person's life; someone who can be flexible and caring enough to listen to the need at hand, whether it be a need for support, for information, for help to articulate and clarify feelings, or merely to have someone listen to the story.

In many instances the person may not know what he/she needs. As caring/healing companions, our task is to listen deeply for the need, in whatever way it is expressed, and be present to that. A person at the end of life, or at any time, for that matter, is not helped towards healing if they need and expect one thing and we offer another. The questions for the healing companion are, "Can I be flexible enough and knowledgeable enough and caring enough to be there as this person needs me right at this time? Can I stand positively powerless with this family member or patient in their powerlessness, stand present with them in their weakness and vulnerability?"

PART 2

In the second part of this paper, I want to reflect with you on the needs of the caring/healing companion–How to take care of self; i.e., how to cope with constant exposure to raw pain and struggle and make a shield that's not a barrier.

The following six suggestions are intended to stimulate your own reflection and insight into ways you, the reader, can enhance your own care for yourself.

1. *Be reflective.* Learn from experiences. The greatest challenge in caring for those at the end of life, is that we, as care-givers are confronted with our own pain and bewilderment and unresolved griefs. The more incapable we become of bearing our own suffering, the easier it is to avoid the suffering of others. Acceptance of

our own feelings and honestly reflecting on and dealing with our own issues, helps us become more compassionate and courageous in our caring for the dying. We need to reflect on our own issues, helps us become more compassionate and courageous in our caring for the dying. We need to reflect on our own experiences and feelings, our "success," as well as our "failures." We all like to be successful, but success does not stimulate growth as much as failure does. What is required of us in life is growth towards wholeness, not success. We must trust that what feels like failure can be a powerful learning moment. This is what keeps us moving and growing as companions (vs. stagnant and stoic in service).

Sometimes, there's just no more room to let someone else's pain in, and as reflective care-givers, we need to get away, recreate ourselves and empty space for others. If we are blind to our own needs, we cease to be helpful to another.

2. *Highlight moments of breakthrough.* Breakthroughs are not necessarily easy and joyful moments. Showing a willingness to be with people when they're in utter despair and need to rage about it can be helpful in breaking through the locked-in feelings of the dying person or family member. This may be a breakthrough, a cathartic moment, that calls for notice and celebration. Persons facing the end of their lives may often withdraw because they do not know what to do–this causes even greater suffering, as indicated above. They need a caring person who is not afraid to stand with them in their withdrawn feelings–and to be allowed to do that may be a step forward for the person, a step that may enable them to touch their pain and begin to speak about it. ("If you press the emotional pain, the linguistic juices will flow.") As a caring companion, note the breakthrough and be content with the person's pace.

3. *Unhook projections and dismantle transferences* on to the helpee. When we "project," we attribute to another a repressed feeling of our own. When we "transfer," we act out of an old emotional reaction to another person who reminds us unconsciously of another significant person from the past. Knowing ourselves and noting our reactions can be invaluable in recognizing and dealing with projections and transferences. We need to separate person from the one he/she reminds us of, as well as to note reactions and feel-

ings that get triggered in ourselves in relationships. When we, as companions, feel ourselves "hooked" by the issues or expectations of a patient, it behooves us to take note and work to understand the message for us, as well as the consequent choices available. Otherwise, we risk being over-burdened and burned out.

4. *Watch out for Messiah complex.* This shows up in an attitude of "mother hen," one that communicates: I am here to "save" this person, to take away their suffering, to solve their problem. Many of us get into caring professions because we want to help. This easily sets up expectations–puts pressure on others to change. Unconsciously, we may act out: "let me help you with your problem and out of your terrible situation." This is not only not respectful of the person's dignity, it is not helpful in bringing the person towards inner freedom. Rather, it keeps them dependent, not self-reliant, and not "in-charge" of their present concern. As caregivers, we need to frequently ask ourselves, "To whose need am I responding–mine or the patient's?"

5. *Come with nothing, but a full nothing*, rather than an *empty nothing.* A full nothing is pregnant with life, with hope, with expectation. It is an attitude of attentive presence to self and to the person being ministered to, but with the clear eyes of faith that say you cannot really help this person, except to be there while God helps them and they help themselves. A full emptiness can be the conduit of God's grace. And if emptiness is full enough, then presence will remind people that God is there (without God-talk). "If you have been to the desert and meet God and become empty, then people come to you, and your presence is healing" (Nouwen, *The Way of the Heart*). When I feel burdened down with peoples' tragedies I've learned that I don't have to work at intercessory prayer. I can sit in God's presence, without packing up a brief case and going to prayer with it. I can let go and release someone to God's care with faith that God cares for this person even more than I do, or than I ever could. Through an exercise of faith imagination I can leave the person resting in God's light, surrounded by God's protection; then I can let go peacefully. As care-givers and healers, we do our best, but a part of that best is realizing how little depends on us.

Another important aspect to keep in mind is the readiness and openness of the dying person to receive help and care. We may be both full of desire to help this person and rich in skill to do so, but we are not mechanics, fixing a machine. We can do nothing without the person's choice. In *Who Dies*, Stephen Levine writes, "When you are working with seriously ill patients, it is important to remember that it is not you who has to do anything. All you have to do is get out of the way so that the appropriate response to the moment can manifest itself. You don't have to save anyone except you. Working with the dying is work on yourself" (p. 167).

6. *Find good companions*. It is essential to find good team members or colleagues, persons with whom to share and process your experiences, especially those that are disconcerting and those that "stick" long after the encounter has ended. Good companions can offer vital help in unhooking projections and transferences, as indicated above, and in helping us objectify what is transpiring. This in turn, helps us be more present and available to both ourselves and the persons to whom we minister.

Good companions also keep focus on all the above needs of caretakers. Clearly, ours is a ministry where we cannot depend on seeing results. We need to acknowledge and compensate for this legitimate need if we are to survive in this journey of caring for people at the end of life.

PART 3

Having reflected on some basic needs in the healing companion, I would like to return once more, to the needs of persons at the end of their life, and offer a list of summary needs of the person at the end of life. As indicated earlier, this is often a time of loss, confusion and crisis. Their need may be for comfort, touch, presence, listening, privacy, support, encouragement.

- They need someone to sit in the mess with them, and break it into manageable pieces.
- They need to be treated as persons, a living person who happens to be dying, and not just a diagnosis.

- They need hope, a refocussed hope which looks at what can be done:–finish business, pain free, legitimize feelings. Many will find hope in the willingness of friends, care-givers to treat them as real persons, whose physical functioning and competency may be impaired.
- They need help to articulate feelings, and to be specific about these. If these remain general and diffused, the dying person cannot make a very orderly assessment about self, because life feels chaotic. If focussed he/she can grasp and confront this crisis better.
- Sometimes unrealistic fears can be explained and eased, but a good deal of suffering has to be lived through, and their need is for someone to sit patiently with them in silence as Job's friends finally did. The very pain itself may lead to resolution or a new vision.

It is an awesome and holy mission to accompany another with care and compassion at the end of his or her life. That we should stand by, wait and pray with the dying and their grief-stricken family members, that we should be among the last to give him or her a drink, or a gentle stroke of the hand or head! This is holy ground indeed, and blessed are we when we take off our shoes and stand with them.

Competency:
The Asceticism of Our Time–
The Role of Pastoral Care
in Ethical Decision-Making

Daniel G. O'Hare, PhD

The same two decades which mark my involvement with the medical world are also two decades which have chronicled the most rapid and expansive development and application of technology, ostensibly in the promotion of health and the service of human well-being. Dramatic decreases in infant mortality and childhood diseases, greater control over formerly catastrophic illnesses, and remarkable advances in both quantitative and qualitative post-disease survival due to the rapid sophistication of antibiotic therapy and the perfecting of new and complex surgical procedures are but a few salient examples of the medical milestones–or, perhaps in a more familiar jargon, miracles–which we now often quickly and unreflectively take for granted. Most assuredly, these comments are not meant to suggest an attitude unsupportive of the continued efforts of medical technology to gain new footholds in the often precarious ascent to the conquering of disease and the improvement of the quality of life.

But the period of the same two decades–and only slightly earlier in medical history–has also frequently witnessed a movement from attending sickness and death to a greater ability to extend the former and to stall the latter, a movement which can, on occasion, quantitatively protract that which cannot be qualitatively improved, a movement which can result in assaulting rather than attending

Presented at Religion and Cancer: A Vision for the '90s.

111

sickness unto death. Quite simply stated, the crux of the ethical quandary which surfaces in that context is merely because something is possible in the framework of the ever-broadening sophistication of medical technology, is it–or should it be–simultaneously ethically indicated? Just because we *can* do something, *ought* we do it? Is it possible, at least on occasion, that failure to address that central question, in all the guises it adopts in the medical arena, can result in a misuse, if not an abuse, of that technology? And is it possible that what is done ostensibly in the name of humanity can result in an affront, a grievous indignity, to the very personhood it is presumably intended to serve? Does technology and its possibilities serve its artisans, its employers, and its consumers; or, metaphorically, do we have a tiger on leash?

While it is true that some ethicists of the "arm chair" variety have made themselves about as welcome–and just as productive–as you would find broken glass in the bottom of your swimming pool, there is yet a function and purpose to ethical reflection which is properly grounded in both an appreciation of the needs and concerns of health care consumers and the goals and possibilities of the medical enterprise. For I suggest that what *can* and, moreover, what *should* be asked is how regularly and how perceptively we have reflected on the human issues and questions generated in the application of medical technology. If unheeded–or, in a more concerted fashion, ignored–are we thereby subtly suggesting that questions of human dignity, the preservation of individual autonomy, respect for personal freedom, encouragement of corresponding responsibility, and the avoidance of duress and manipulation simply do not exist or are morally neutral? Does even the suggestion of the need for reflection on, but not necessarily control of, the management and utilization of human and economic resources forged into medical technologies strike only a discordant note?

Have we unwittingly created by inattention or indecision allowed to flourish a "circular fallacy?" Dimly aware of, although not necessarily more educated in, the previously untapped possibilities of medical technology, has society, in turn, demanded more of it? Has a once unquestioning and largely untutored medically lay population grown, especially through media coverage of more celebrated cases–more news on more medical possibilities in more startling fashion everyday–more presumptive concerning the potential of that technology? Have we thereby vested medicine with an authority and a responsibility beyond its expertise, an expertise that we are only too willing to vehemently condemn, or threaten with costly litigation, when it apparently fails us? And, indeed, what has come to be viewed as failure? Have sound technological aspirations genuinely collapsed, or are there immutable limits rather than periodic hurdles over which the technology may not pass? Has our reflection, both lay and medical, on the human and ethical implications of the application of that technology been either consonant or conversant with its development? Or has the mandate–born of confusion, hope, and even denial–simply exacerbated our demands on the medical world, demands which even as they are addressed only further goad our individual and corporate presumptions? How often and how willingly are we able to do a reality check on the circularity, thus created, of the charge made to medicine? At what point has it so transcended the current or reasonable future possibilities of medical technology as to render the process specious?

And what of the medical world itself? Has not the response to the possibilities of medical innovation and the increasingly critical demands of consumerism been that of a technological imperative? Because it *can* be done, it *should* be done, with the possibility of its *being done* subtly taking precedence over other considerations. What may not have been even imagined in a previous generation, what medicine did not presume nor was challenged to approach, has now become accomplished fact in our midst. But such "accomplished facts" are also, with an alarming regularity, being brought to the courts and to the theological and philosophical communities for evaluation. We now have the technology to manipulate nature from before conception to after flat EEGs. What is often unclear and what raises the specter of ethical compromise, what we need to attend to, is whether that manipulation is by invitation or invasion of that process.

What I am concerned about, what I feel you should be concerned about, is the role of pastoral care in the ethical issues which are thus raised in medical care and treatment. Far from being a morose preoccupation with the morbid or somber, my involvement in the medical arena and with those who are sick and dying has lent a freshness and vitality to my experience of living and, in the communication of that vitality, a liberating sense of urgency and immediacy in prioritizing the issues and questions of life. It has also been a labor not completely devoid of humor. I am reminded of my grandfather and his best friend. Both gentlemen were quite elderly when I came to appreciate them. My grandfather's friend was an undertaker, and, every year at Christmas, my grandfather would receive a card from his undertaker friend signed, "Eventually yours!" I hasten to add that my grandfather–perhaps solely out of spite–managed to outlive his friend.

But as is painfully obvious to each of us, there are human dreams associated with sickness and death which are anything but humorous and appear to be even devoid in hope. It is precisely in that context that I began what I now recognize as my interest in the ethical problems associated with medicine. I would appreciate being anecdotal, and there is something I should explain. I am not only Doctor O'Hare. I am also Father O'Hare, a Jesuit priest, and much of my previous involvement in medicine has been in the area of pastoral care. In that "incarnation" I came to recognize not only the need for ethical reflection but the role–and the potentially critical role–of pastoral care in facilitating the discussion of and suggesting a resolution for issues at the confluence of medicine and morals.

From the first day on the floors, now many years ago, as an aide in a terminal cancer hospital, I was forced to confront my abysmal ignorance as I urged a patient to close his eyes for the woman who I thought was bathing him. Only when she explained to me that he was dead did I realize how foolish I appeared. All the good will in the world notwithstanding, I simply did not know *what* was transpiring. If we are ever going to offer assistance or deign to comment on the quality of someone's care and, in so doing, seek credibility, we have to first understand the context in which we presume to speak. I was convinced that I could handle the situation, but I was so wrong. Who would have sought my opinion later that day? Who would have believed that I had any basis, any right, to suggest anything? We need to know *what* it is we are talking about.

Not long after attempting to talk to–to offer "instructions" to dead bodies–I found myself speaking with an elderly woman admitted from a city hospital. Diagnosed as terminally ill with cancer, she had been literally and figuratively triaged to less than appropriate care. She arrived filthy, disheveled, and in great pain. As I started to comb her hair, she began to scream, and her head, my hands, and the mattress beneath her were suddenly filled with blood. She had not been cared for in so long that in the sweat-producing heat and pain which she had experienced, the pins in her hair had rusted, become attached to her scalp, and I was ripping them out as I ran a comb through her hair. That quickly brought the attention of the professional staff, but, as I stood there, transfixed by the horror and rendered impotent by my crushing sense of guilt for the pain which I had unwittingly, but no less really, occasioned, I found myself muttering "No one, *no one* should die like that!" Why had that happened; why was that allowed to happen? Thus while it is important to know "what" is happening before we attempt to comment on it, it is also important—as moral agents—to ask the question "Why?" Why would anyone think that was adequate or professional care? Why should someone be subjected to such a physical assault and such a personal affront? Why should those who find themselves suffering from a physically deteriorating disease also be victimized by psychological debilitation at the hands of those who chose to do less when doing more was so in order? Why was it that an inability to cure resulted in an apparent unwillingness to care?

It is—and unfortunately but finally understandably so—in the eyes of some health care professionals nothing short of a most brazen hubris for non-medically savvy individuals to dare to inquire into—much less question—their competence or authority. Yet to every medical professional willing to engage in the discussion, to those I have taught and to those with whom I have worked, I have addressed two questions. Depending upon one's response to either or both, the entire course of care for an individual and his or her family will be designed accordingly.

I offer for your own reflection the following: First, is the subject of attention, the object of care, a disease site, a lesion, or a tumor which now only circumstantially happens to inhabit the body of an individual, or is it—or should it be—an individual who now only circumstantially is plagued by or the victim of some medical anomaly? Secondly, is there any human condition which of necessity does not transcend the compartmentalization of being merely and completely physical or solely and exclusively medical? If that is the case, can even the *accumulated* insight of any single field of human understanding stand equal to the task of addressing or eliminating the difficulty?

Depending upon one's response to the first question—whether one is the caregiver, the care receiver, or even the care observer—either fairly unbridled liberty in the ostensible pursuit of healing disease is permitted or, from the outset, a respect for the individual and the unique facets of his or her personality which weigh heavily in relation to the medical problem is assured. The rhetorical nature of the second question is underscored in observing the final frustration—to patients and loved ones alike—which can result from inadequate care which was destined to be such from the outset because less than was possible, less than was essential, in both understanding and appreciating the many levels of concern of the individual patient was taken into account. What extra-medical factors—personal, familial, social, cultural, religious, and even economic factors—must be included in the most inclusive care of any individual?

If there is any benefit to be derived from being confronted by a barrage of "hard medical cases," it may be to alert and, in alerting, to heighten our consciousness of the complexity of some medical-ethical dilemmas and the perplexity involved in attempting to resolve them. That a moral voice is in order is becoming more acceptable if, indeed, not more actively sought.

But whence this moral voice? From whom and in what context may we presume reflection, deliberations, and decisions which flow from sound moral reasoning? While lack of formal ethical training is no immediate indication of moral ineptitude, to remain uninformed is to face the context of moral decision-making with a fragile consistency. It is also not automatically the case that exposure to moral and ethical principles (autonomy, self-determination, beneficence, non-maleficence, informed consent, and confidentiality) assures probing and satisfying solutions to moral dilemmas. What is fairly self-evident, however, is that if informed deliberations and decisions can be in error, to engage in uninformed or untutored responses is to court disaster. And in the case of pastoral caregivers, it is, for patients and their families, to court the possibility of unmitigated disappointment for those who have chosen to place their implicit trust in their religious representatives.

Therefore, I would suggest that one such voice in framing ethical questions may be that of pastoral care but if and only if it is, indeed, a voice which concertedly proposes and echoes sound moral principles. For an assertive voice, even a persuasive voice, is not necessarily a moral voice. Can we permit the reaction of "outraged common sense," frequently little more than masked prejudice to suffice? Even as those who may well have had the longest or the most recent and thorough training in ethics, the fundamental problem of the pastoral caregiver in the medical arena is–and may well remain–credibility.

Even within my own religious polity, I can speak with little more than provisional authority. But I am secure in my presumption that the abuses discovered therein were not of our making alone. The most ecumenically sensitive suspicion is that no one religious polity has managed to corner the market. For reasons which escape my ability to comprehend–much less justify–resulting in disservice to all parties concerned, in the not too distant past we regularly assigned to hospital ministry–in an era preceding accredited and accrediting clinical pastoral education programs–individuals whose only recommendation was that they had proven largely unsuited for any other ministry. Individuals frequently in need of care, certainly of companionship, and critically short of stability, individuals who were both emotionally fragile and physically depleted were stripped of community supports and, often without having their own issues addressed, were expected to function twenty-four hours a day in an atmosphere for which they were ill-prepared and which was singularly anxiety-producing. That they often met with tremendous difficulties or proved unsatisfactory should have come as no surprise. Yet, they were there, ostensibly they were available, but who was going to be well served by their interventions, especially in matters as weighty as medical-ethical decision-making potentially involves? Who was going to view them as either comfortable or conversant with the field in which they operated? Who would grant them a hearing regarding their opinions of morally or ethically indicated procedures? Credibility is a problem. Veils and collars and titles may well produce deference, but deference is not credence! Competence may well be the asceticism of our time for pastoral caregivers. An ability to remain current with the issues and questions of the field in which they chose to labor, especially as the same issues are informed by reference to specific religious creeds, is absolutely essential for the contemporary pastoral caregiver. I can make my assertion no more strongly than to state that ethical decision-making cannot be relegated to the markedly well-meaning but the radically uninformed!

Pastoral caregivers need to reflect on moral issues. They need to understand or at least recognize areas of potential ethical compromise. They need to be sensitive to the relationship between those questions and the needs of the individuals to whom they minister. Do they take time–are they willing to make time–to examine their own inclinations, feelings, and prejudices and so attempt to educate them? Or are they willing to pander with pious platitudes? Can we afford spiritual pablum where the diet is so rife with moral and ethical controversy? How prepared is today's pastoral caregiver to insert himself or herself into the morass of medical-ethical decision-making? How current is such reflection in light of contemporary theological or philosophical perspectives?

I cannot belabor the point too long or too strongly. If pastoral caregivers are to insert themselves–and the insertion is at least theoretically possible *and* necessary–into the circle of ethical decision-making, they must do it as professionals. Advances in credibility are often made only slowly and painstakingly and can be vitiated rapidly. Credibility necessitates a proper orientation to the environment to maximize experience and reflection on that exposure. If pastoral caregivers are genuinely fearful of that space–physical and psychological–and permit that discomfort to control their responses, or if they are unheedful of the critical time that the present moment could be in the lives of those they serve, their credibility suffers, if not vanishes, accordingly. They need to have done their homework approaching that environment and the consequences of remaining there, and they need to continue to do their homework to function viably.

While credibility is an absolutely essential preliminary to contributing as a pastoral caregiver to ethical decision-making in the health care setting, there are other factors in the pastoral dimension of care which, when properly utilized, can place the pastoral caregiver in an advantageous position in dealing with the patient and the family and even the balance of the health care team. Not least among those factors in the pastoral relationship is that wherever and whenever a positive relationship exists between pastoral individuals and those receiving their ministrations, it is characterized by an attitude of deep trust and confidence. This can be of critical importance to the individual arriving more often than not unwillingly in the sterile, unfamiliar and foreboding environment of a hospital, those who arrive faced with the sudden onset of disease, or the prospect of protracted suffering, or the imminent reality of impending death. It is precisely the pastoral caregiver who may be best able to assist in that transition, representing as he or she does the security and stability of a relationship known and appreciated outside of and prior to hospitalization.

The merit of that bond of trust is twofold. To the patient it can provide reassurance and invite openness, thus permitting the patient a sounding board for fears and anxieties; while for the patient it can provide advocacy and the potential for adequate representation of questions and fears regarding treatment and rehabilitation or disability and death. Without betraying or compromising the confidentiality which can be invoked as a cornerstone of this relationship of trust, the advantage to the total care of the individual is in the acknowledgement that not everyone is hearing the same things from the same person. In helping the patients to frame their questions, unfold their fears, and delineate their hopes in the security of a relationship which purports to contend with ultimate issues, the pastoral caregiver is able to bring, at the behest and with the permission of the family, the patient's own desire for information and contribution to the decision-making process. *Who* is saying *what* to *whom*?

It is, or should be, in the nature of the pastoral care relationship that it is simultaneously committed and objective, striving for open and honest communication between and among all parties to the decision-making process and, indeed, facilitating that process where fear and a sense of intimidation have inhibited dialogue. These are not covert strategies for undermining the power or authority of all those who rightfully must be included in ethical decision-making. Rather they constitute a rationale supporting the presence of pastoral care in that decision-making process if, in fact, it is a voice which lends interest and assures support for the individual patient.

The greatest benefaction of the pastoral caregiver to the entire health care picture may be that activity of bridging gaps, illuminating the distances which can obtain between individuals who are, in the hands of fate, tossed together. A caution to be introduced into that imagery is only that bridges exist to span chasms. The labor of the pastoral caregiver is fraught from the outset if their ministrations serve only to broaden that abyss. The pastoral caregiver has no less than a moral imperative to both personally respect and professionally promote the dignity of the person and to strive to inculcate that same attitude of respect in others, particularly those whose expertise will be sought by people in their need. You can challenge, but you also need to support. You can learn to ask not only *what* is being done but *why*. You can encourage openness and strive to discover, from as many vantage points as possible, what is hoped, what is feared, what is sought by individuals, and, therefore, begin to address what would be the most correct way, the moral way, of responding to those concerns. You have a great potential, and to the extent that you present that potential as a viable component in ethical decision-making, the reality of patient care may be altered. Theoretically, pastoral care always has a voice in addressing the total needs of the patient, but practically speaking it is a voice which will be sought only as it is recognized as credible. Pastoral care represents one of the few functions within the health care environment which is recognized, understood, and even appreciated outside that environment; and thus the pastoral caregiver has the potential for immediate access into the cares and concerns of the lives of patients. Pastoral care therefore has the possibility of developing–and rapidly–rapport. You can be perceived as worthy of trust, remembering only that trust is difficult to achieve, easy to lose, and more arduous to regain. Where faith–faith in God, you, or what you represent–is a salient feature of the individual's life, your counsel will be sought, your opinion respected, and your advice followed. But there is a corresponding responsibility to be both compassionate and competent. Thus the role of pastoral care, especially in the manifestly complex field of medical ethics, is no place for the well-meaning amateur.

Yours can be a posture of freeing, lifting the loneliness of isolation and fear from those who suffer while attempting to free care-givers from the often unrealistic burden of the demand to heal. It is finally possible that your task, your privilege, your moral responsibility, is to assist others in rendering fully and freely to God what is already in God's hands.

Cancer Care and Community Clergy: Hospital Based Training Models

Mark Peterson, MDiv

This year in Florida alone, sixty-eight thousand people will have the opportunity to have the bombshell dropped on them: "You have cancer." How many times does that happen across the country? One million, forty thousand. Heart disease strikes more often, but is not quite as frightening. Cancer scares people.

Cancer is the second most common cause of death in the USA. In any congregation of people, twenty-five percent will develop cancer. Of that group, half will be cured, and the other half will die of their disease. The clinicians say that if people would simply take advantage of *existing screening, diagnostic, and treatment methodologies*, the cure rate would jump from fifty to seventy-five percent–twenty-five out of every one hundred people who develop cancers die needlessly! Given this alarming statistic, the clergy of this country need to expand their concern for their congregations. It is no longer enough to focus only on souls. Clergy must be concerned about bodies, too. This begins with education–first the clergy, then the congregations they serve.

THE HISTORY–THE RATIONALE

Cancer Residency for Clergy began in 1975 under the direction of Chaplain Lowell Mays at Madison General Hospital in Madison, Wisconsin. It was co-sponsored by the Wisconsin Division of the American Cancer Society. For ten consecutive weeks, four clergy at a time came on Sunday afternoons and stayed day and night through Wednesday. During that time they were exposed to basic information and the latest trends in cancer diagnosis and treatment.

There was room to accept forty clergy. Four hundred applied! The program was deemed a smashing success. The students loved it because they had been given a chance to see the inner sanctum of a hospital and had all their questions answered. Hospital administrators loved it because they believed in education and were able to make unparalleled public relations contacts with important community leaders. The American Cancer Society loved it because they had been able to educate a caregiver population they had not reached before, namely, the clergy. It was not long before the National American Cancer Society heard of this exceptional program and presented the program with its highest honor, the National Honor Citation. The word began to spread.

Now, fifteen years later, twenty-one hospitals around the country offer Cancer Residencies for Clergy (by state):

State	No. of Programs
Arizona	1
Delaware	1
Florida	6
Nebraska	1
New York	1
North Carolina	1
Ohio	3
Pennsylvania	1
Wisconsin	6

(Specific centers are listed in Table 1. The local American Cancer Society office or the author may be contacted for more information.)

The American Cancer Society went a step further in 1989 creating a National Work Group on the Clergy and Cancer Care. The author is privileged to serve as this group's chairman. The mission is two-fold: (1) To educate clergy to be better pastoral caregivers to cancer patients, and (2) To foster educational and service programs in congregations.

TABLE 1. Cancer Residency for Clergy (4/91)

Chaplain Gail Wade
Scottsdale Memorial Hosp-N
10450 N. 92nd Street
Scottsdale, AZ 85261
602-860-3000

Rev. Lloyd Evans
Medical Center of Delaware
P. O. Box 6001
Newark, DE 19718
302-733-1000

Rev. Al Hall
University Hospital
655 W. 8th Street
Jacksonville, FL 32209
904-350-6515

Rev. Luther Jones
Jackson Memorial Hospital
1611 N.W. 12th Avenue
Miami, FL 33136
305-549-7260

Rev. David Diercks
Orlando Regional Medical Center
1414 S. Kuhl Avenue
Orlando, FL 32806
407-841-5111

TABLE 1 (continued)

Rev. Clarke Mundhenke

Lincoln General Hospital

2300 S. 16th Street

Lincoln, NE 68502

402-475-1011

Rev. Gib Mueller

Director of Pastoral Care

Geauga Hospital

13207 Ravenna Road, Rt. 44

Chardon, OH 44024

216-286-6131

Rev. Wesley Manfalcone

Martin Memorial Hospital

P. O. Box 9010

Stuart, FL 34995

407-287-5200

Rev. Donald Bane

Westchester County Medical

Center

Valhalla, NY 914-285-7123

Rev. Mark Peterson

Bayfront Medical Center

701 6th Street South

St. Petersburg, FL 33701

813-893-6623

Rev. Dan Campbell

Moffitt Cancer Center

P. O. Box 280179

Tampa, FL 33682

813-972-4673

Chaplain Lewis Lint

Pitt Memorial Hospital

108 Martinsborough Road

Greenville, NC

919-551-4100

Rev. Dwight Baldwin

Mory Rutan Hospital

205 Palmer Avenue

Bellefontaine, OH 43311

513-592-4015

TABLE 1 (continued)

Rev. Kenneth Eggen

La Crosse Lutheran Hospital

1910 South Avenue

La Crosse, WI 54601

608-785-0530

Rev. Larry Karls

707 South Mills Street

Madison, WI 53715

608-251-6100

Rev. Don Corbin

St. Charles Hospital

Navane Avenue

Oregon, OH

419-698-7378

Chaplain Lynwood Swanson

Pastoral Care Service

Fox Chase Cancer Center

7701 Burholme Avenue

Philadelphia, PA

215-728-2944

Rev. George Robie

Sacred Heart Hospital

900 W. Clairemont

Eau Claire, WI 54701

Deacon Earl Charlier

St. Vincent's Hospital

P. O. Box 1221

Green Bay, WI 54305

414-433-0111

Rev. Lindy Nelson

St. Joseph's Hospital

P. O. Box 1221

Green Bay, WI 54305

414-433-0111

The latter goal exists because overall forty-five percent of the population of this country regularly attends worship services. In rural areas the percentage is even higher. If people could be reached in the context of their faith communities with the American Cancer Society's important message of prevention and early detection, lives will actually be saved.

STARTING A CANCER RESIDENCY FOR CLERGY

Step One. To begin a Cancer Residency for Clergy (CRC) program, one first should attend one elsewhere. There is no better way to get a grasp of the program or to decide whether an institution is capable of providing the requisite faculty and facilities. Prior blessings from the administration and influential members of the medical staff whose practice is heavily populated with cancer patients is also quite helpful because their active support will be necessary later.

Step Two. The hospital's ability to meet basic program requirements needs to be assessed. All of the following questions should be answered "Yes":

- Does the hospital have a designated cancer center, floor, or unit?
- Does the hospital offer radiotherapy?
- Does the hospital have an active surgery schedule (fifteen or more cases/day)–some of which are cancer related?
- Is the faculty available to present all mandatory topics on the curriculum requirements list (Table 2)?
- Does the hospital have more than one chaplain?
- Is someone available to do case review if the five day program is offered?
- Can the hospital offer housing to clergy residents?

If any of the above questions were answered "No," a co-sponsorship of a CRC program with another health care institution might be considered? Such partnerships often work nicely, bypassing barriers based on competition.

Step Three. After development of a potential faculty list, the half day (three hour) version of the program can be offered. The local

Table 2. Clergy Education Programs/Cancer Residency for Clergy American Cancer Society, Florida Division Inc.

<u>Curriculum Requirements</u>

<u>Mandatory Topics</u>	<u>Suggested Presenter</u>
<u>One Day Programs:</u>	
1. What Is Cancer?	Pathologist
2. Cancer Diagnosis - By Radiology	Radiologist
3. Cancer Treatment - By Surgery	Surgeon
4. Cancer Treatment - By Radiotherapy	Radiotherapist

131

TABLE 2 (continued)

Mandatory Topics	Suggested Presenter
One Day Programs:	
5. Cancer Treatment - By Chemotherapy	Hematologist/Oncologist
6. Psychosocial Care of Patients and Families	Social Worker/Psychologist
7. American Cancer Society - What It Is, What It Does.	ACS Unit Staff/Volunteers
Three Day Programs, the above, and:	
8. Pre-Test, Post Test	
9. Pediatric Cancer	Pediatric Oncologist

10.	Pastoral Diagnosis Issues	Chaplain
11.	Cancer Diagnosis - In The Lab (Tour)	Lab Staff
12.	Cancer Diagnosis - By Radiology (Tour)	Radiology Staff
13.	Cancer Treatment - By Surgery (Tour, Surgery Observation)	O. R. Staff, Surgeons
14.	Cancer Treatment - By Radiotherapy (Tour, Lecture)	XRT Staff, Radiotherapist
15.	Terminal Care, Hospice	Inpatient Nursing Staff, Hospice

TABLE 2 (continued)

<u>Mandatory Topics</u>　　　　　　　　　　　　　　　　　　　<u>Suggested Presenter</u>

<u>Five Day Programs, the above, and:</u>

16.　Patient Visitation, Case Review　　　　　　　　Students, CPE Supervisor

<u>Optional Topics</u>

1.　Cancer Treatment - By Plastic Surgery　　　　　Plastic Surgeon

2.　Cancer Treatment - By Bone Marrow Transplant　BMT Unit Staff, Medical Director

3.　Cancer Research　　　　　　　　　　　　　　M.D., PhD Research Staff

4.	Pediatric Psychosocial Issues	Pediatric Social Worker
5.	Health Care Costs	Finance V.P.
6.	Ethical Issues in Cancer Treatment	Chaplain
7.	Care of the Caregiver	Chaplain, Psychologist
8.	Ronald McDonald House Tour	Volunteer, Staff
9.	Hope Lodge Tour	Volunteer, Staff

American Cancer Society will probably be happy to serve as a cosponsor. Speaker presentations and clergy interest can then be evaluated.

The following format might be used:

Length	Speaker	Topic
10 min	Chaplain/ Administrator	Welcome
30 min	Pathologist	What Is Cancer?
20 min	Radiologist	How Is Cancer Diagnosed?
60 min	Panel: Surgeon Radiologist Oncologist	How Is Cancer Treated?
15 min	Break	
20 min	Social Worker/ Psychologist	Psychological Issues
10 min	Chaplain	Pastoral Issues
15 min	ACS Staff or Volunteer	American Cancer Society Resources

For those based in congregations, this type of program or a portion of it is ideal for adult education–either as a single event or a series. The local ACS will supply speakers. Some people will be too shy to attend a lecture or too afraid to make an appointment with a physician. So, displaying ACS tracts and leaflet in the church narthex will allow them to read and maybe help themselves. Materials on the following usually have the greatest impact:

Lung Cancer
Colo-rectal Cancer
Prostate Cancer
Breast Self-Examination

Those four are also the most treatable and/or preventable.

Step Four. Throughout the country, area representatives of the national ACS will assist in obtaining the latest materials (outlines, sample forms, letters, learner objectives, etc.). If these cannot be reached, however, the national telephone number in Atlanta is 404-320-333 (the Service and Rehabilitation Department).

A Final Thought. When a CRC program is offered, students, hospital administrators, and the American Cancer Society all love it. But the most important group of all, the people in the pews, become the real beneficiaries when a pastor, priest, or rabbi becomes cancer literate. They benefit because they receive better pastoral care from a trained clergyperson who will be helping them take better care of themselves. And an even greater gift than that will be given–some of them will even live a little longer.

Index